THE TERMINAL PATIENT: ORAL CARE

THE TERMINAL PATIENT: ORAL CARE

EDITED BY

AUSTIN H. KUTSCHER,

BERNARD SCHOENBERG AND ARTHUR C. CARR

With the editorial assistance of

Lillian G. Kutscher

Published by

THE FOUNDATION OF THANATOLOGY

Distributed by

COLUMBIA UNIVERSITY PRESS

New York and London 1973

Originally Published in the
Journal of Thanatology and
the Archives of the Foundation of Thanatology
by the
Health Sciences Publishing Corp., 1972

Copyright © 1973 The Foundation of Thanatology
ISBN: 0-88238-701-4
Library of Congress Catalog Card Number: LC 72-9892
Printed in the United States of America

FOREWORD

Traditionally, the primary responsibility for the definitive care of the terminal patient rests with his physicians. It is becoming more and more apparent, however, that the comprehensive care of such a patient requires a team of specialists in order to treat all of the manifestations of terminal illness as they present themselves in the various regions of the body. When the oral cavity is the site of a specific complication, those with specialized expertise in the treatment of this crucial area should be recognized as having significant roles to play. The doctors — general practitioners of medicine and dentistry, internists, surgeons, radiotherapists, psychiatrists — as well as the supporting personnel — nurses, dental hygienists, clergymen, social workers, psychologists, and others — should be prepared to perform whatever terminal care procedures are deemed to be advisable.

All doctors and their supporting staff will encounter the emotional problems of the dying patient and his family, the problems of care per se, as well as their own personal and emotional interactions in the contact with death and dying. In large measure, the general responsibilities will not differ significantly from caregiver to caregiver; in specifics they *must* and *do*. It is the purpose of this book to introduce the essence of the sum total of the oral care problems which will be encountered and for which solutions must be attempted by all who give care to the terminally ill patient.

Among those health professions acknowledging and delineating the psychosocial and general care problems faced by terminal patients and their families is the profession of dentistry and its allied personnel. The extraordinary importance of the mouth to the dying patient makes imperative the need for maintaining all of its structures in the best possible condition and for providing a degree of comfort that will permit the patient to live out his days with a minimum of discomfort and a maximum of dignity.

Frederic P. Herter

I share with many the obvious thought that death must become a topic for a great deal more contemplation by all human beings and by those concerned with health care, in particular. It is a very germane topic and, perhaps, a point of immediate departure in contemporary planning for the health of our citizenry. In many circumstances, we must give care to patients throughout the course of illnesses even when there is little or no hope of being able to interrupt the disease process.

During the past 25 years, the breakthrough in information and the ability to give care toward goals of curing many disease entities have been fantastic. Those in the health professions have been criticized by patients and others for a seeming detachment from the philosophy which guided them during the period which preceded World War II. At that time we appeared to be serving to give care and support, while now we appear to be absent. Because more cures are possible, more are expected; and more and different types of care are also expected not only by the professionals themselves but also by those to whom the care is given. We use words like "continuity of care" and "cure." Yet we realize that these are goals which are often hard to attain. If we think of the individual in terms of his total health and the responsibility of the health professional in every discipline to care continuously in the effort to reach the goal of helping each individual maintain and sustain an optimum level of existence in contradistinction to concentration on cure, some of our efforts may be more successful.

We must talk and share our knowledge. We must readjust our focus so that at those times when we cannot give the gift of healing, we can still add enrichment to the quality of life for our patients and their families.

Helen Pettit

PREFACE

The need for care efforts in treating the oral complications of the terminal patient highlights dramatically the need to train all professionals in accepting a role in the life of these patients. It is now evident that proper terminal care can be approached only by a willingness on the part of all caregivers to invest the patient's final days with dignity.

The mouth of the terminally ill patient often provides the final means for him to communicate with his environment and the last organ for expressing and receiving pleasure. Its care during the terminal phase of life requires skilled and understanding forms of therapy, a routine of maintenance which can restore and support self-esteem, dignity, physical comfort and esthetic integrity for the patient. If oral tissues and facial contours are affected and altered by disease, all untreated psychological-physiological complications can disrupt and disturb most distressingly the patient's relationship with his family and his professional caregivers.

To bring the oral problems of terminal patients into focus — and to integrate educational and motivational efforts toward their solution by the dental practitioner and his professional colleagues, the physician, the nurse, the social worker, the psychologist and other allied health team members—a joint commitment was made by the Foundation of Thanatology and the School of Dental and Oral Surgery, Columbia University, Columbia-Presbyterian Medical Center, New York, New York. This volume contains the papers presented before this unique conference.

A wide range of questions involving the oral care of the terminal patient is dealt with by the chapter authors from psychosocial as well as pragmatic points of view. The need for new approaches to the oral care of the dying and innovative methods of dealing with the grieving and bereaved family is stressed. Such topics as the following are examined in depth: the behavior and attitude of the physician, dentist and nurse when caring for a terminal patient; the problem of providing active therapy as well as adequate pain relief for those painful oral problems which may beset the terminal patient; the importance of speech preservation; psychopharmacotherapy and its effects on mouth comfort, disease and speech; oral prostheses and their associated problems for the terminal and/or declining geriatric patient; nursing and dental hygiene care; responsibilities of the social worker toward the patient and his family; proper treatment for the terminal pediatric patient; and so forth.

The Appendix of this book presents a case history of a patient afflicted with an oral malignancy from which he suffered for 16 years. The salient features of this particular case exemplify further, and epitomize, the aspects of oral disease which may be the locus of the cause of death and/or as the unwelcome accompanying complications appearing in patients dying from other than a stomatologic disease: oral hygiene, nursing care, medical specialty care, oro-medical care, psychiatric and psychopharmacologic care, restorative dental care, surgical care, "routine" dental care, geriatric care—and in this case the psychosocial contingencies inherent when a man's normal instrument of communication is attacked and virtually destroyed by disease, impaired by treatment and afflicted by the sequelae of local malignant deterioration and/or local effects of distant nonstomatologic causes of death.

A strikingly ironic note is added by this example to the philosophy of caring for the *oral* problems of the terminal patient. It can certainly be concluded that oral care should and can be expanded far beyond the limited dimensions of "ordinary" dentistry.

A.H.K., B.S., A.C.C., L.G.K.

The editors of this book are members of the faculty of Columbia University. Dr. Austin H. Kutscher is Associate Professor and Director, New York State Psychiatric Institute Dental Service, School of Dental and Oral Surgery, Columbia University, Columbia-Presbyterian Medical Center, New York; and President of the Foundation of Thanatology. Dr. Bernard Schoenberg is Associate Clinical Professor, Department of Psychiatry; and Associate Dean and Director of Allied Health Sciences, College of Physicians and Surgeons, Columbia University. Dr. Arthur C. Carr is Professor of Medical Psychology, Department of Psychiatry College of Physicians and Surgeons, Columbia University.

All royalties from the sale of this book are assigned to the Foundation of Thanatology, a tax-exempt public research and educational foundation dedicated to education and research efforts in studying the psychosocial problems inherent in dying, death, loss, grief, and recovery from bereavement.

CONTENTS

Foreword
 FREDERIC P. HERTER
 HELEN PETTIT

Preface

OVERVIEW

Psychosocial Aspects of Oral Care in the Dying Patient
 BERNARD SCHOENBERG AND ARTHUR C. CARR 3

A Philosophy for the Oral Care of the Dying Patient
 AUSTIN H. KUTSCHER 16

The Oral Cancer Patient with Terminal Disease: The Patient, the Family, the Doctor and Death
 ALFRED S. KETCHAM 24

Oral Care of the Dying Patient
 S. GORDON CASTIGLIANO 31

Hermes and Beyond
 IAN W. D. HENDERSON 52

The Oral System in *Bereavement*
 DAVID PERETZ 68

SELECTED MEDICAL SPECIALTIES

MEDICINE

Internal Medicine and the Oral Care of the Dying Patient
 MANUEL OCHOA, JR. 77

RADIOLOGY

The Radiotherapist's Relationship to the Dying Patient
 HARRY L. BERMAN 92

NEUROLOGY

Oral Care of the Dying Patient: Neurological Aspects
 THOMAS J. BRIDGES, JR. 99

CHEMOTHERAPY AND PHARMACOLOGY

Cancer Chemotherapy: Implications for the Dentist
  SUSAN MELLETTE 106

Psychopharmacological Agents, Narcotics, Analgesics and
  Oral Problems of the Dying Patient
  EDWARD H. MONTGOMERY AND FRED F. COWAN .. 112

Psychopharmacological and Analgesic Agents Employed in the
  Terminal Care of 78 Oral Cancer Patients
  IVAN K. GOLDBERG, AUSTIN H. KUTSCHER,
  BERNARD SCHOENBERG, HARVEY GRALNICK AND
  HARLAN A. KUTSCHER 143

PEDIATRICS

Oral Care of the Terminally Ill Child
  ALBEN B. CURTIS 150

Management of Oral Problems in the Dying Child
  MARTIN I. LORIN 156

DENTISTRY

Dentistry and the Dying Patient
  PAUL SCHEMAN 162

Dental Care for the Terminally Ill Patient
  M. B. QUIGLEY AND I. L. SHANNON 167

Maxillofacial Prosthesis
  NORMAN G. SCHAAF 173

Dental Care of the Dying Patient
  CLIFTON O. DUMMETT 178

Dental Needs of the Chronically Ill and Disabled Aged:
  As Seen by the Dental Hygienist
  GEORGIA HALL 184

NURSING

Postoperative Nursing Care of Head and Neck Patients
  ALICE COSTELLO 190

Nursing Care and Interpersonal Relationships
    MADELAINE A. BADER 195

SOCIAL WORK

Oral Care of the Dying Patient: A Social Worker's Point of View
    EVELYN F. COOPER 208

The Social Worker's Role in Care of the Dying
    CONSTANCE LAMB AND ELIZABETH R. PRICHARD .. 214

PASTORAL CARE

Pastoral Care of Patients with Oral Cancer
    ROBERT B. REEVES, JR. 228

APPENDIX

Oral Cancer Surgery Notes: Care of Sigmund Freud
    FROM ERNEST JONES 235

Contributors 255

Index
    ELAINE A. FINNBERG 259

ACKNOWLEDGMENTS

The authors wish to acknowledge with deep gratitude the encouragement given this project by Melvin L. Moss, D.D.S., Ph.D., Dean of the School of Dental and Oral Surgery, Columbia University, New York, New York and Lawrence C. Kolb, M.D., Chairman of the Department of Psychiatry, College of Physicians and Surgeons, Columbia University, and Director, The New York State Psychiatric Institute, Columbia-Presbyterian Medical Center; and further express appreciation for the dedicated efforts of Professor Helen Pettit, Professor Elsa Poslusny, Professor Constance Cleary, Professor Roberta Spagnola and Miss Ann O'Donnell of the School of Nursing, Columbia-Presbyterian Medical Center; Miss Linda Draper and Mr. Steven Gross of the Psychiatric Institute Dental Service staff; and Mrs. Ruthann Zanis, Mrs. Betty Loshin, Mrs. Priscilla Hawkins, Mrs. Blanche Grieco, Miss Elaine Finnberg, Mrs. Rafaela Lorenzo, Mr. Harlan Kutscher, Mr. Austin Kutscher, Jr., Mr. Martin Kutscher and Mr. Richard Goldberg working on behalf of the Foundation of Thanatology.

Special recognition is also extended by the authors for the assistance and guidance of Leon Lefer, D.D.S., M.P.H., M.D.

OVERVIEW

Psychosocial Aspects of Oral Care in the Dying Patient

Bernard Schoenberg* and Arthur C. Carr*

Case Summary

The patient under consideration was a male Caucasian physician who died at the age of 83. Over the previous period of 16 years, the patient, following initial radical surgery for the removal of a cancer that extended from the right side of his jaw across his palate, underwent 33 documented surgical procedures. The entities which required further surgical and other modalities of intervention until the time of his death were multifocal areas of leucoplakia, various precancerous proliferations of tissue, and finally frank recurrent carcinoma.

He had noticed the original "leucoplastic growth" himself and had self-diagnosed it as an epithelioma. He, nevertheless, waited two months before seeking consultations with other physicians. At that time he was told by a dermatologist that the lesion was a leucoplakia due to smoking and was advised that a "very slight operation" was necessary to remove it. Suspicious, the patient then consulted with a close friend and asked him for help that he might "disappear from the world with decency" if he was doomed to die in suffering. A further concern was for his elderly mother who, he felt, would not be able to cope with his dying—if that was to be the case. The friend reassured him that the lesion was truly leucoplakia.

The patient then presented himself to a distinguished surgeon at an outpatient clinic which was part of a general teaching hospital which had no private facilities. The operation did not go as had been expected and so much blood was lost that the patient was put to bed in a small room already occupied by a cretinous dwarf. Profuse bleeding ensued, and the patient could neither speak nor call out. The dwarf summoned help and, perhaps, saved his life. The next morning the surgeon demonstrated the patient as a case study to a group of medical students before he was permitted to go home.

---

* Department of Psychiatry, College of Physicians and Surgeons, Columbia University, New York, New York

The excised growth was submitted to the pathology department as a biopsy. The specimen proved to be malignant but the patient was not told this.

The surgeon had not taken various precautions against the shrinking of the scar so that considerable contraction occurred which greatly reduced the size of the patient's mouth opening and which caused considerable hardship thereafter.

The surgeon's attitude had been cavalier. Perhaps he was under the impression that he had done everything possible and that the growth could not recur. Or, on the other hand, he may have regarded the case as hopeless. Two X-ray treatments and a series of drastic treatments with radium followed. The patient suffered greatly from the latter's toxic effects for months.

At almost the same time, a beloved four-year-old grandchild died following a tonsillectomy. The patient said that this loss killed something in him for good and he became very depressed and seemingly indifferent towards the threat to his own life.

He had continuous discomfort from the scar over a period of months. A physician friend, upon examining the area, noticed what he believed to be a recurrence of the growth and indicated the necessity for its removal. But the patient still was not told the serious nature of his lesion because there was concern over whether or not he would consent to the surgery since his mourning over the death of his grandson seemed to have deprived him of the will to live. His family and friends were consulted regarding the decision of whether or not to tell him that the lesion was malignant. It was decided not to tell him. He did consent to further surgery.

Shortly thereafter, another unmistakably malignant ulcer in the hard palate which invaded the neighboring tissues including the upper part of the lower jaw and cheek was discovered. Two extensive operations were then performed by an eminent surgeon—under local anesthesia.

Years later, when told of the discussion and of the decision, he demanded, with eyes ablaze, "By what right?" However, he admitted that from the beginning he was sure that the growth was cancerous. It is not evident exactly how or when or by whom he was eventually told the true diagnosis.

There followed 16 years of distress and pain, interrupted only by recurrences of the disease and further operations, radiation treatments, cauterizations, devitalization of teeth, etc. In addition, he developed a heart "condition" and abdominal complaints—which seemed to concern him more than did his mouth cancer.

The intra-oral prosthesis (an obturator) made for him was practically impossible to remove or insert because he could not open his mouth widely enough. He described it as "the monster." A second and third prosthesis were made but with only slight improvement. Speaking and eating were also practically impossible, his speech was markedly affected; damage was done to the Eustachian tube, as the result of constant infection in the area over the years—which caused a marked hearing impairment on one side. Throughout the years, the discomfort and pain in his mouth became almost unbearable. At one point he sought consultation with an eminent surgical prosthodontist who was visiting near him. At first the man refused to see him. Finally, he did and worked for 20 days on the prosthesis, which still was not satisfactory; charging the patient, now nearly bankrupt, $6,000. On many occasions, and for long periods of time, he was forced to stop seeing his own patients with a resultant precipitous decline in his income. However, he always insisted on paying his own physicians.

In discussing his situation in later years, the patient found it particularly hard to forgive those who had kept the whole truth from him. What he seemed to have minded most was the implication that he might not be able to face courageously a painful truth, since he considered his ability to do so one of his outstanding virtues.

At his own request he underwent surgery for bilateral ligature of the vas deferens on both sides hoping that sterilization might alter the course of the cancer. Orthoform, topically applied by his daughter throughout the night, proved to help the pain for some years, but its continous application led to a local keratosis, and therefore its use had to be restricted.

Six years after the first surgery, an internist, who had been analytically trained, was engaged to supervise his general care. At their first interview the patient laid down one basic rule—that the truth should never be kept from, however painful it might be. They shook hands on this, and the patient added: "I can stand a great deal of pain and I hate sedatives, but I trust you will not let me suffer unnecessarily."

He had been a heavy cigar smoker but abstained from time to time because of his heart condition only. But, at the age of 74, he decided that abstinence was no longer justified and resumed smoking.

Fifteen years after the original surgery, during a course of radiation therapy, it was discovered that the metal in his prosthesis was producing secondary radiation and another had to be built. At this time, also, what he called the most severe surgery since the first operation was performed. He never recovered fully postoperatively and became more frail.

Shortly thereafter, other lesions were observed. The surgeons decided that these were inoperable and incurable and that only palliative treatment should be attempted. For a short time the patient actually appeared to respond favorably. However, he wrote to a friend, "I am not getting on well; my complaints and the effects of the treatment share the responsibility in a proportion I cannot determine. The people around have tried to wrap me in an atmosphere of optimism: the cancer is shrinking; the reactions to the treatment are temporary. I don't believe any of it, and don't like being deceived."

He refused all medication except aspirin. The odor from his wound became so offensive that even his favorite chow dog shrank from him—a most disturbing event to him.

He kept getting weaker and weaker; finally, he said to his internist, "... you remember our first talk. You promised me then you would help me when I could no longer carry on. It is only torture now and it has no longer any sense." He displayed no emotionalism nor self-pity, only reality.

The following morning his physician gave him 1/3 of a grain of morphine. He was so weakened that he fell asleep. The next evening he died.*

The patient's name, of course, was Sigmund Freud.

The problems related to death and dying in our culture, particularly those most relevant to the oral management of the dying patient, are

---

*Extract prepared by and quoted with the permission of Lillian and Austin H. Kutscher, based on material in *The Life and Work of Sigmund Freud*, Vol. III, by Ernest Jones. New York: Basic Books, 1957.

highlighted by the history of an individual whose search for the truth throughout his professional career provides a model that might well be emulated by all scientists, particularly those interested in a study of the care of the terminally ill.

In our culture death has unfortunately been treated traditionally as a taboo topic, generally to be avoided, and only in the last decade has it become a subject of scientific interest and investigation. Ross (1), Feifel (2), and others have described their initial difficulties in gaining access to terminal patients, as well as the anxiety of hospital personnel in allowing scientific study of the dying process at a time when, as Gordon Allport (3) has indicated, young scientific investigators feared that an interest in a "taboo" topic would "blight their professional careers." Many investigators (Feifel, Ross, Weisman and Kastenbaum (4), Glaser and Strauss (5), Saunders (6), and others) have now demonstrated, however, that no untoward effects result from dealing with death candidly and that, to the contrary, it may have a therapeutic effect.

The changing attitudes we are evidencing in relation to the study of death and dying can be equated with and are similar to the changes brought about largely through Freud's influence in relation to the topic of sex. The heightened scientific interest in death and dying during the past decade perhaps has not been adequately explained. Is the current interest in death related in part to the threat of nuclear holocaust, the disintegration of familiar social institutions, the threat of violence, dire predictions concerning over-population and environmental pollution leading to extinction? Or is it related to our more recent confrontation by youth with its emphasis on the integrity of the individual? No single explanation seems to suffice. Concurrent with increasing willingness to deal candidly with death and dying, however, recent rapid technological developments in medicine which can prolong life indefinitely are raising serious moral, ethical and social issues. Questions related to organ replacement, organ repair, euthanasia, "life in the test tube," genetic counseling, sex determination, renal dialysis, etc., lead many to assume that death is possibly no longer inevitable and that man has an increased control over life.

In this context the physician's efforts may become directed towards an heroic struggle with disease and death rather than the quality of the individual's existence. While the patient initially may be reassured with the energetic determination of health personnel to rescue him, once he recognizes his incurability he seeks more humane considerations such as communication, warmth, continuity of human interaction, respect and efforts to maintain dignity and intimacy rather than the heroic measures which frequently prevent what is referred to as a "safe" or "dignified" passage.

Cicely Saunders who founded St. Christopher's Hospice in London in 1967 chose the term *hospice* after careful thought. The term, meaning a resting place for travelers, represents the values and philosophy of the institution which is a hospital for the terminally ill. Dr. Saunders (7) writes, "We can only prepare the path the individual has to travel. Our aim is to handle our treatment so that pain and distress are quieted and our patients are enabled to remain themselves, able to find their key to the treatment as they see it and to use that key in their own fashion. We have no doubt that they are going through an experience that has meaning and that what we see is not just the long defeat of living but a positive achievement of dying." The majority of patients are usually referred from other hospitals and larger medical centers where they have already undergone extensive surgical, radiotherapeutic and chemotherapeutic treatment, but may have several more months left to live. Surgical procedures, intravenous solutions, blood transfusions and experimental procedures or drugs are avoided at St. Christopher's. Recognizing that cure is unrealistic, the administration and staff of the hospital are oriented towards a philosophy of offering comfort and relief. The staff, once it gives up the battle for cure, becomes identified with an approach that emphasizes living rather than dying.

Dr. Saunders differentiates between prolonging living and prolonging dying. She states "Because something is possible does not mean it is necessarily either right or kind to do it" (8). To realize that the patient is dying is not a defeat on the part of the patient or the doctor. Dr. Saunders feels that this recognition indicates respect and awareness of the individual person and his dignity. Heroic measures when a person is in a terminal stage are usually neither for the patient's nor for his family's benefit.

It is, of course, because of the family's or the doctor's anxiety about death that dying generally is not discussed openly with the terminally ill patient. Feifel (9) has noted that, just as was true with Freud, "Most seriously ill and terminally ill patients generally prefer honest, plain talk from physicians and family about the seriousness of their illnesses. They want to voice their doubts, affirm their faith, and communicate what their pending separation means. They do not want their problems ignored or reassurances they perceive as falsehood." Eighty-two per cent of Feifel's patient sample wished to be informed of their condition. He postulated, based on his observations, that one of the major factors influencing certain physicians to enter medicine is "to govern their own above-average fears concerning death."

Contemporary American culture with its emphasis upon youth, vitality, materialistic success and the denial of death has had a profound impact upon practicing health personnel. Cure is given much greater value in the medical profession than is comfort. Cure has become associated with success while the death of a patient has become equated with failure.

The degree of the avoidance of death in the medical profession is best illustrated by a survey of a group of hospital interns and residents who were graduates of 15 medical schools. Not one of the group could recall having been instructed during their medical school education on the requirements for the diagnosis of death (10).

Evidence presented elsewhere by the authors (11) documents the failures in medical and nursing education to provide students with adequate training in the care of the terminally ill and the bereaved. For example, results indicated that about 50% of the faculty respondents to the survey of medical schools reported that the requirement for the diagnosis of death are not formally included in their medical school curriculum. Over one-third report that the physician's responsibility in the care of the bereaved is not included in the curriculum. About two-thirds report feeling only *somewhat pleased* or *displeased* with the teaching efforts to prepare medical students for the care of the dying patients. In spite of this dissatisfaction, only one-third of the respondents indicate they plan to make any curriculum changes with regard to the care of the dying patient.

Students canvassed reported feeling that discussions related to controversial issues associated with the care of the dying patient such as euthanasia, definitions of death, ethics of organ transplantation, addiction of terminal patients to narcotics, etc., are frequently absent in the medical, dental and nursing students' curricula. About two-thirds of the students felt it desirable that their school make curriculum changes with respect to teaching the student how to care for the dying patient.

Specifically relevant to the oral care of the dying patient, a more recent survey eliciting responses from 108 deans and chairmen of departments of 38 dental schools reveal such results as the following:

Almost two-thirds (63.6%) report that the dentist's responsibility in regard to the oral care of the terminal patient is not included in the dental student's curriculum, while slightly over one-half (51.4%) indicated similarly regarding the oral care of the terminal oral cancer patient.

More than two-thirds report that they are less than very pleased or moderately pleased (10.3% and 14.0%) with their teaching efforts to prepare dental students to provide oral care for the terminal patient or for the terminal oral cancer patient, respectively.

Approximately three-fourths (76.6%) reported that their school does not regularly assign students to provide dental care for patients suffering from a condition which may lead to death.

Over three-fourths indicate that when students are given examinations they are rarely (38.3%) or never (40.2%) asked questions about their role in the oral care of terminal patients, while almost two-thirds indicate that they are rarely (37.4%) or never (24.3%) asked questions about their role in the oral care of the terminal oral cancer patient.

The most frequently checked reason (42.1%) for why these matters (care of the dying patient and discussions with the patient's family before and after the patient's death) are not considered in the dental school curriculum was that of *lack of curriculum time*. The least frequently given reason (13.1%) was *lack of student interest*, suggesting that all other given reasons—lack of faculty interest (28.0%), lack of personnel (33.6%), lack of relevance during this period of education (34.6%) and lack of printed subject matter or teaching materials (24.3%)—have priority over the student's interests.

Surveys of fourth year students of two dental schools support the contention that too little emphasis is placed on the oral care of either the terminal patient or the terminal oral cancer patient in their training. Consistent with the reported views of faculty members, lack of faculty interest is given more frequently as the reason why care of the dying patient is neglected than is lack of student interest.

In the sensitive task of providing care for the terminally ill, students obviously need not only emotional support from training personnel, but also a model of how ideal psychosocial care should be given. At a time when most college students are coping with anxiety related to death by repression and denial, the health professional student is confronted with death as a fact of life and is expected to deal with it effectively and remain emotionally accessible to the severely ill or dying patient. Many students find this a formidable task and some can only cope with the problem by shutting out their own emotions and by becoming inaccessible to the dying patient. Emotional withdrawal, avoidance and isolation with emphasis on tasks and ward rituals become the means of decreasing anxiety in order to maintain stability. Unfortunately, such early experiences become the prototype for the student's later relationships with patients.

Probably the most demoralizing and devastating experience for the dying patient is the experience of isolation leading to greater fears of abandonment. The isolation is increased by the poor communication between the dying patient, the doctor and other health professionals and members of the family. This is developed in large part through the emotional and physical inaccessibility which those surrounding the patient utilize as a defense against their own feelings of helplessness, anger and grief.

The enforced dependency of terminal illness also leads to feelings of weakness and defectiveness and arouses feelings of humiliation and shame, leading to anger, guilt and depression with a loss of self-esteem. With the feelings of guilt and depression, the chances for pleasure and gratification are reduced considerably. Accompanying these feelings are always the developing feelings of grief as the patient recognizes in fantasy the losses he will suffer, the loss of loved ones especially. The process of dying for the patient implies pain, loss of control, deterioration, helplessness, dependency, humiliation and abandonment.

A recent report by Klagsbrun (12) describes an experiment in self care undertaken by the patients of the cancer ward in a hospital. The patients' morale was increased considerably when they were permitted to see themselves as productive human beings. Before the program could be undertaken, the nurses were assisted in handling their feelings in regard to terminally ill patients. The nurses harbored angry feelings towards the medical staff for lack of emotional backing and support in helping them deal with terminal patients. In the program, patients were urged to take passes and leave the ward. They requested to be involved in various projects such as sewing and artwork and generally were pushed toward activity. The patients made their own beds and would get their own water and ice. Before long, they were taking water to the bedside of those who were too sick to care for themselves. After a while, they took over the linen closets and made up beds for very sick patients. A communal dining room was established to provide a nucleus for socialization and normal living. These activities tended to break down the isolation that some patients suffered and to decrease the loneliness. Patients "discovered a new communal strength that came from shared experience." Before long, they organized evening activities and showed slides of their travels. When patients who had remissions left the hospital and returned, a not uncommon reaction was a sense of relief at coming back to a setting that regarded them with expectations. They immediately entered into increased activity and appeared happier. It would appear that as much attention is required towards improving the quality of the patient's life during the terminal stage as might be **devoted** to pain-relieving drugs or psychopharmacological agents. All of these factors should be seen as a continuum in which the patient is afforded the greatest degree of comfort and the largest measure of dignity.

There is perhaps no aspect of patient management that serves as a better model for what ideal psychosocial care represents than that of the oral care of the dying patient. The mouth is an especially vulnerable organ, particularly in illness (and in aging itself) when regression often occurs. As indicated elsewhere:

"The mouth is generally recognized as the first area of gratification. The lips, tongue, and buccal mucosa are erogenous zones of the body and throughout life are associated with pleasure as well as self-preservation, love, hate and destructive impulses. The infant's view of the surrounding world is determined by his early mouth relationships, usually with his mother. The oral cavity can easily become the area of displacement from other parts of the body and the zone for expression of unconscious feelings.

"Psychoanalytic investigators have consistently noted the significance of orality in depression and have related early childhood disappointments in love to the propensity for depression in later life. Freud compared depression (melancholia) to normal grief, recognizing that some patients have a predisposition, related to early life experiences, to react with depression when confronted with loss of loved persons or valued objects. He described the process as a regression to the oral stage of development . . .

". . . The mouth is commonly regarded as an instrument of attack, reflected in such expressions as "sharp," "biting," or "cutting" tongue.

"The oral cavity, as an erogenous area and a body orifice, readily becomes a zone of displacement from other parts of the body. Psychoanalytic studies and investigations of dreams indicate that bleeding from the oral cavity may be unconsciously experienced as menstruation, abortion, sexual invasion, rape, castration, and death. (13)."

Quite apart from any symbolic significance the mouth may have in general, in terminal non-oral illness such problems as mouth odor, soreness, pain and dryness, disturbances of chewing, swallowing and speech functions, reduction in salivary flow and alteration in salivary composition occur and add directly to the feelings of dependency and loss of self-esteem which accompany any illness. For the health practitioner, these problems challenge the patience, ingenuity and dedication of even the most skilled and experienced worker.

In the management of the terminal oral cancer patient, even more serious difficulties exist. Common problems to be confronted include facial and mouth deformities, fungating uncontrolled cancer tissue with concomitant mouth odors, inability to articulate and speak properly and the total failure of all other mouth functions. Certainly no more poignant report of the kind of difficulties which oral cancer may elicit can perhaps be found than Freud's recognition that even his dog was shrinking from him because of the offensive odor of his cancer.

Furthermore, the diagnosis of cancer always carries with it the threat of death for the patient. This fear in the patient is magnified by the fear with which cancer is viewed by the layman and health professional. Other diseases which may carry an equally serious threat to the biological existence of the patient and which may be less amenable to treatment are frequently approached with less apprehension.

The word "cancer" invariably evokes thoughts of an eroding, devouring and mutilating illness. Quite speculatively it might be suggested that while fear of death gains its magnitude partly because of the fear of the unknown, death may also represent essentially an oral threat, the fear of being eaten. Certainly for the primitive man death did present the very realistic threat of being eaten. This fear may be reflected today in the burial customs which encase the body in presumably impenetrable casements to protect it forever against predators. Perhaps then, for this reason, our conception of cancer as a devouring illness concretizes what really underlies the fear of death which is so prevalent in all mankind.

Whether or not this speculation is true, feeling about the threat of cancer often exerts its damaging effect long before the patient seeks medical assistance and may contribute to an unfortunate delay in seeking treatment, with such denial frequently resulting in death. There is the suggestion that denial operated even in Freud who delayed seeking consultations with other physicians until two months after his initial difficulties first became apparent to him. Although there are no research studies on physicians as dying patients, many clinical observations indicate that physicians may deny extensively the significance of their own symptoms or illness, in spite of their academic knowledge and medical training.

The practical problems of oral care confront the health professional with what perhaps is one of the greatest challenges in caring for the terminally ill. The degree to which the patient achieves gratifications, maintains self-esteem, communicates his fears and desires, expresses gratitudes and dissatisfactions, and is offered what Weisman labels "safe conduct" (14) depends to a large degree upon maintenance of good oral care. It is hoped that what follows in this volume will provide some guidance, support and direction in terms of how this can be achieved.

References

1. E. Ross, *On Death and Dying*, New York: Macmillan, 1969.
2. H. Feifel, "Death," in N. L. Farberow (Ed.), *Taboo Topics*, New York: Atherton Press, 1963.
3. G. Allport, "Foreword," in N.L. Farberow (Ed.), *Taboo Topics*, New York: Atherton Press, 1963.
4. A.D. Weisman, and R. Kastenbaum, "The Psychological Autopsy: A Study of the Terminal Phase of Life," *Community Mental Health Journal*, Monograph Series No. 4., 1968.
5. B. Glaser, and A. Strauss, *Awareness of Dying*, Chicago: Aldine Publishing Co., 1965.
6. C. M. Saunders, "The Management of Patients in the Terminal Stage," in R. W. Raven (Ed.), *Cancer*, London: Butterworth, 1959.
7. C.M. Saunders, quoted by Sister Zita Marie Cotter in "The Care and Understanding of the Dying," *Archives of The Foundation of Thanatology*, *1* (No. 2): 14, 1969.
8. C. M. Saunders, "The Moment of Truth: Care of the Dying Person," in L. Pearson (Ed.), *Death and Dying: Current Issues in the Treatment of the Dying Person*, Cleveland: The Press of Case Western Reserve University, 1969.
9. H. Feifel, "Death," in *Taboo Topics*, edited by N. Farberow, New York: Atherton Press, 1963.
10. J. D. Arnold, T. F. Zimmerman, and D. C. Martin, "Public Attitudes and the Diagnosis of Death," *Journal of the American Medical Association*, *206*:1949, 1968.
11. B. Schoenberg and A.C. Carr, "Educating the Health Professional in the Psychosocial Care of the Terminally Ill," In B. Schoenberg, A. C. Carr, D. Peretz and A. H. Kutscher (Eds.), *Psychosocial Aspects of Terminal Care*, New York: Columbia University Press, 1972.

12. S. C. Klagsbrun., "Cancer, Emotions and Nurses," *American Journal of Psychiatry, 126*:1237, 1970.
13. B. Schoenberg, A. C. Carr, A. H. Kutscher, and E. V. Zegarelli, "Chronic Idiophatic Orolingual Pain," *New York State Journal of Medicine, 71*:1832, 1971
14. A. D. Weisman, "Psychosocial Considerations in Terminal Care," In B. Schoenberg, A. C. Carr, D. Peretz and A. H. Kutscher (Eds.), *Psychosocial Aspects of Terminal Care.* New York: Columbia University Press, 1972.

A Philosophy for the Oral Care of the Dying Patient

*Austin H. Kutscher**

The Terminal Condition

There comes a time in life when a complex of symptoms appears, a diagnosis is made, and an unfavorable prognosis is pronounced. Except in instances such as acute myocardial infarction or cerebro-vascular accidents, human life then enters a period of terminality and thenceforth follows a prolonged downhill trajectory (often requiring hospitalizations), which is accompanied by increasingly debilitating physical conditions, organ system failures, emotional turmoil and perhaps a comatose state from which the patient lapses into death.

It is a truism, usually repressed, that from birth onward man is in a terminal condition and each day brings him closer to his death. In actuality, there are varying degrees of terminus. (A symposium solely to discuss the semantics of the words "terminally ill" and "dying" might be of great value, even of necessity.) Cancer patients surviving surgery may not be free of disease and may require palliative care by radiotherapy (or vice versa) and thus survive for many additional years, even though they are never "cured." Can they be considered among the "dying" patients during this extended period? Chemotherapeutic agents also can be utilized to give them a longer lease on life when malignancies recur and are either inoperable or unresponsive to radiation. Is this another stage of terminality? These are but two examples of the problem of defining terminality, but there are many more.

The cardiovascular patient or the stroke victim can survive a series of coronary occlusions, cardiac arrests or major and minor strokes. Intensive care, medications, ever-improving surgical and nursing techniques and electronic and mechanical devices have favorably changed the response of many failing hearts and altered the course of circulatory ailments.

So our practical definition of "terminal" also changes from day to day, and we are forced to include not only the hospitalized patient who may linger for days, weeks or months, but also the patient whose

---

*School of Dental and Oral Surgery, Columbia University, New York, New York, Director, New York State Psychiatric Institute Dental Service, New York, New York.

symptoms are for a short or long period "under control," who is discharged from the hospital and for that period often continues to function as a member of a social schema. Thus, broadened theoretical and psychosocial definitions of the word cause us constantly to consider the priority of care for the so-called "terminal patient."

The Dentist, the Medical Team, and the Dying Patient

In a sense, most patients are under the care of a "team," although this is scarcely noted formally. Unfortunately, two of the principal team members—the physician and the dentist—often do not share that part of working together for the welfare of the patient which they should. In many instances, both have had similar exposure to the basic sciences in their respective medical and dental schools, but their pathways diverge and the one becomes a doctor involved with the functioning systems of the human body while the other, all too often, becomes a doctor who limits the direction of his talents to the tooth and its supporting hard and soft tissues and, likewise, limits his medical responsibilities to the patient to the bounds of his operatory. The patient's teeth, often almost apart from the rest of his mouth, are then cared for as if the care rendered and sought had no connection with any other part of the human being under treatment.

The average dental practitioner would, at first thought and in all honesty, say, "I have never treated a dying patient." But how many of these same practitioners have not done some form of rehabilitation on patients with congestive heart failure, women who have survived mastectomies but are *not* free of disease, patients on renal dialysis units, patients with advanced arteriosclerotic brain disease, patients with cystic fibrosis, patients with advancing chronic emphysema, and many others? Emotionally and intellectually, he establishes semantic blocks against the word and concept of the "terminal" or "dying" patient in order to achieve the results (even to the point of perfection) for which his training has so properly motivated him. Except for those dentists who have a hospital affiliation, the dentist avoids treating the bedridden patient who is on a downhill course. Even if the dentist is available physically and emotionally, he is generally never given the opportunity to be part of the team that should include the physician, the dentist, the nurse, the dental hygienist, the chaplain, the social worker and others—all of whom can play important roles by their attendance to the dying patient at various stages.

Realistically speaking, few dentists are motivated to treat the hospitalized dying patient. Priorities have been established by a pattern of dental education which changes only slowly. Several classes of students may graduate before newer concepts are introduced into the curriculum.

Questions are also raised about patient priority and training priorities for the dentist. Whom should he treat? What should his motivations be? Should he treat the young child, the young adult, the middle-aged, whose life spans have a normal expectancy? Should his energies and talents be "wasted" in giving comfort to the geriatric or the dying patient? According to a recent survey, the dentist in his four years of dental school, rarely, if ever, sees or treats a dying patient—at least not knowingly by many of our definitions of "terminal" or "dying." Adding further to this unfortunate picture, there is often no economic gain from the hours to be spent with dying patients, nor professional satisfaction if the dentures he has labored over have to be delivered to the funeral parlor.

It should be added that medical schools are hardly blameless, since the orientation of the medical student is based on death denial and an emphasis on defeat of death. It took the advent of such advances as heart transplant surgery to force the establishment of *ad hoc* ethics committees to seek definitions of "death" itself so that one patient is not killed in order to save another. Likewise, new devices have provided the potentially heroic measures now available for the prolongation of dying—not living—and have created situations where it seems evident that at some point a decision must be made "to pull out the plugs" and let the patient die.

Concern for the Dying Patient

As the tides of education change, the health professional of the near future will be guided by a deeper concern for his patient as a total individual, molded by a social environment and community, pressured by unique emotional stresses, by successes and failures, by gains and losses—including the loss of body parts and self-image, of significant loved ones, and eventually the prospect of loss of his own life. The lines of communication among all the health professionals must multiply so that one discipline will learn from the others and share with the others not only knowledge, but also the care of the living *and* of the dying patient.

Until some ten years ago, except by a rare physician, medical concern for the dying patient was limited to fending off death, with only a secondary regard for the emotional comfort of the patient. The patient was given physical care but little or no psychological support during his terminal days. Only in recent years has it become apparent to medical personnel that dying is a phase of living and that the patient, though near death, is still a sentient human being. Regrettably, dental concern for the dying patient still remains almost nonexistent in most institutions. Few nursing homes provide dental care but most do have paramedical personnel who understand only that dentures should be cleaned occasionally and not switched from patient to patient.

Yet the dentist is beginning to acknowledge that he is a member of the health team which is interested in and concerned with allowing the patient to live his final hours in comfort and dignity. Although the dentist doesn't sign a death certificate, there is no doubt that his education and early training should reinforce his awareness of the fact that he is treating a whole human being, not just a tooth. He must also be made to feel that his obligations do not end when the patient walks from his office but extend, as do the physician's, to the deathbed.

New Trends in Education

Dental education is being supported in this philosophy by the clinical cancer training programs introduced and financed by the National Institutes of Health to train students in every aspect of this disease—this training extending beyond the traditional exposure to the subject in the dental-medical curriculum. The dental student has never before had an opportunity to become acquainted with the bedridden patient. Yet this exposure is still too limited. It is true, of course, that not every dentist wants to be involved in or to some degree specialize in giving this kind of care. From the dental classes of 40 or so students at the School of Dental and Oral Surgery, Columbia University, all of whom during their third year take a cancer training course, it would be gratifying if two elected to spend a part of their professional careers in clinical and research efforts directed toward caring about and caring for the problems of the dying.

Most graduate dentists now serve in internship programs where hospital dental facilities exist. Yet many such health care institutions do not provide dental care services for the hospitalized patient, let alone the dying patient. These men are not trained to work on institutionalized people of any description. The financial problems concomitant with such an extension of oral care facilities into hospital settings are beyond the scope of this discussion. However, the hospital which serves as a center for community health care should have as a member of its staff a dentist capable of functioning at the patient's bedside as a member of the health team.

Examples of Oral Care Opportunities Related to the Dying Patient

The physician has not in fact been trained to treat oral problems. Generally, he avoids the mouth, examining only the tongue and the throat. Yet rarely does he call upon a dentist to ease the discomfort of the patient whose oral tissue resistance to moniliasis has been lowered by the administration of antibiotics or whose salivary gland function has been reduced by the use of phenothiazines, tranquilizers or radiation. Physicians do not really recognize what the dentist can do to help their patients. Nor are they truly aware of the extent and intensity of oral complaints. They are concerned with the treatment of other body regions and the dentist for them is less than a secondary figure. Nor does the physician realize that the patient may have preoccupations with his mouth, high in the hierarchy of his suffering and from which he is suffering unnecessarily.

The maintenance of proper oral hygiene is left to the nurse or the dental hygienist (in the rare hospital that has such), and they perform as best they can to make the patient comfortable in this regard. The instances where the whole dental team is involved are pitifully few, in spite of the fact that there are problems of the dying patient which a dentist and proper dental therapy can alleviate. Ill-fitting dentures can be replaced or refitted by quickly made or relined temporary prostheses; the electric toothbrush can be used by a weak patient or held for him by a nurse or hygienist or even a family member so that the mouth can be freshened and kept moderately clean. So far no substitute for natural saliva has been found and little effort is being expended to devise such a compound, yet some attempts are being made to develop devices that even the cachectic patient can operate to deliver moisture of such a kind into his mouth.

Examples of the Importance of Oral Care

The mouth of the terminal patient becomes increasingly important to him as his deterioration progresses. The patient who loses coordination and muscle strength of the hands cannot write. The edentulous or the partially edentulous patient or even the patient with a full complement of teeth may suffer from xerostomia, dysgeusia from debris and sordes, mucous solids from saliva which are not easily removed without strenuous mouth movements by the tongue or the ingestion and/or flushing of copious amounts of fluids (such as mouthwashes), or infections, and so lose even the ability to speak properly. How then can he communicate with his caregivers or his loved ones?

If it is not cared for properly, the mouth can become a source of great discomfort not only in the patient who is dying from oral cancer but in those who are dying of cancer in other sites of the body or in patients suffering from chronic diseases. The mouth may remain as the last area of gratification and satisfaction with which the patient may indulge himself—even if only to speak. How many such handicaps, as those listed above, should be permitted to exist? How significantly should the ills of the body be allowed to compound themselves without intervention, especially in the circumstance of *terminal function?* The patient's last days may be very important ones for expressing feelings, for ventilating fears and anger, for expressing love, for relating to an environment that he is no longer a part of.

Conclusions

What can be accomplished must be measured at the present time in terms of limited and restricted goals, but these goals will become in time greatly expanded. The state of the art is such that much can be attempted by exploring for more enlightened and extensive goals, even with the drastic financial strictures now in evidence. In summary, the following suggestions are offered:

1) An emotional groundwork should be laid for the dental student. Initially, this will require basic and adequate instruction in the behavioral sciences. As an adjunct to formal lectures, seminars or open discussions of the emotionally charged topics of dying and death should be held. Through participation in these discussions, inhibitions, fears and insecurities associated with terminal illness can be recognized and dealt with. Psychiatrists, psychologists and other behavioral scientists can be available to monitor such sessions and give support to the dental faculty, the undergraduate and postgraduate student and members of continuing educating courses.

2) The problems confronting the dentist as he tends the dying patient should be examined. The dental student should be brought into the hospital very early in his training so that he can begin to see the patient in the hospital and not just imagine the scene of his possible future work. He should make rounds and discuss the terminal patients. Patients should be seen in all types of situations: ambulatory, in a wheelchair, in bed. Teaching the differential diagnosis of a patient should include a consideration of the patient's whole history; his life style, his hopes and expectations; the specifics of systemic disease processes and their ultimate oral sequelae in the terminal patient; the extent to which such a patient

can tolerate normal procedures; the status of the oral tissues of the dying patient; the obvious medical needs of the patient dying of oral cancer or with cancer invading or metastasizing to the mouth; and an ordering of priorities for his care.

3) The dentist and the physician should assume coordinated and cooperative roles, working together to care for the dying patient. And, in similar fashion, so should the nurse and the dental hygienist. The dental staff should join in the rounds and the discussions involving terminal patients in order to devise a conceptual approach for their oral care and should set up inservice educational programs for all members of the health team.

4) Approaches should be established to accentuate and delineate the best available methods of oral care of the dying patient by the dentist, the hygienist, the physician and the nurse. Each patient is entitled to a complete oral examination and adequate attention to his oral needs. Physicians should be made aware of the fact that oral care is just as important to their dying patients as it is to their vital ones. Routine preventive efforts, often minimal therapy, can prevent the increment of unnecessary oral pain.

5) The nonhospitalized or even hospitalized dying patients should have central community facilities, often existing but seldom utilized, made available and staffed by dentists prepared to treat oral complications. Government agencies must be made aware of the fact that death is a part of life and that obligations for geriatric and terminal patient care do not end when the individual's productivity ends. Lack of money is not a suitable reason nor the only reason for the absence of such facilities: the need for them has been ignored by administrators whose efforts have been directed elsewhere, consciously or in another variation on the theme of denial.

6) Research needs should be postulated and protocols designed so that when funds and personnel are available (and, as is well known, dental research has low priority on the grant-money ladder), extensive dental research may be undertaken without undue delay.

7) Plans should be laid for the future of dentistry wherein the dentist is encouraged to fill a role on the health team, particularly that team *devoted* to the care of the dying patient.

The assumption of leadership is necessary in the early stages of any program. Initiative is required to inform as many influential people as is possible in the health sciences fields of the profound significance of the clinical and psychosocial problems inherent in the care of the still explosively emotionally charged mouth of the dying patient—even though some individuals in positions of authority in hospitals or schools may not be particularly sympathetic to the problems or the care of the moribund. Aroused interest in the dynamics of psychiatric and clinical care problems should produce solutions; all caregivers can then strive to institute the changes needed for the proper oral care of the terminal patient.

The Oral Cancer Patient with Terminal Disease
The Patient, the Family, the Doctor and Death

*Alfred S. Ketcham**

The judgment and wisdom of even the most experienced physician may too often be challenged by the medical and emotional management of the incurable cancer patient when all conventional modes of treatment have failed to produce a positive response. He finds himself involved in handling or "treating" the patient's family as well and may be forced to spend more time in explanation and consolement for them than in the actual care of the patient. Too often, the family's lack of understanding about what is being done, and why one course of action has been chosen over another interferes with the medical attention and care being given the patient. The situation of the pre-terminal and terminal oral cancer patient may be particularly stressful for all concerned because the local tumor and its regional neck metastases may be grossly apparent in all their disfiguring exophytic, odoriferous manifestations rather than hidden in the body or beneath the bed covers. The following discussion will outline some of the considerations which often must be faced and how they might be handled when treating the oral cancer patient who has failed to respond to cancer therapy.

"We Can't Leave Any Stone Unturned"

Whether the patient is being treated in a university research center, a cancer hospital or in a community clinic, he and his loved ones find it difficult at times to accept even the most experienced of judgments. In the hysteria and/or anxiety that accompanies cancer treatment failure, following misguided neighborly advice or frankly fraudulent claims of cure from so-called "cancer clinics" may deplete a family of its economic resources. More importantly, failure often leads to malcontent as the family members try to leave "no stone unturned" in their attempt to offer the cancer victim everything possible towards cure. While family arguments and embitterment may result, it really is the patient who feels the brunt of such misunderstandings. He suffers both physical misery from the treatments imposed upon him and emotional distress as he becomes aware of the turmoil his illness is creating within his family.

---

* Chief, Surgery Branch and Director of Clinical Services, National Cancer Institute, National Institutes of Health, Bethesda, Maryland.

It is the physician's responsibility to act as care-manager and family counselor, even though his advice may have been previously shunted aside. While everyone may be looking for that "one chance in a million" to help the incurable patient, a sympathetic but disciplined and authoritative guiding hand may be all that is needed to pull the family back together and, in so doing, to provide the patient with the comfort and support he needs from those who love him.

Misguided Kindness

Often the terminally ill patient is astonishingly alert and aware of his condition. In some instances, the presence of a tumor mass may be seen in the mirror, felt with the hand or tongue or may impede respiration, swallowing or speech. An attempt to mislead such a patient is misguided kindness and the physician's refusal to acknowledge his own awareness of the seriousness of the problem makes the patient mistrust his medical management. Once he discovers that his doctor has lied to him (it matters not how well intentioned), the breakdown in trust and reliance starts and, often, the initiative and will of the patient to fight for life and to help himself die in dignity vanish.

The patient usually needs to be told only that which is obvious to his eye. Often he will ask little or appear to be unconcerned about the seriousness of his condition. This type of reaction allows a patient the comfort of ignorance and optimistic fantasy. The patient deserves to know what he wants to hear, but the answers to his questions should leave him with the hope of pain relief, tumor regression or therapy response. To lie to the responsible, questioning patient, particularly the adult who has family responsibilities, is truly misguided kindness.

Tumor Dissemination Today, Local Recurrence Yesterday: The Focus of Attack

Not too many years ago, the cancer ward or the terminal care facility always had several patients who were "existing" with large exophytic neck masses or oral facial tumors which were a manifestation of local and regional recurrence following cancer therapy. The unit personnel were attuned to carotid hemorrhage precautions, exophytic tumor debridement procedures, and tracheostomy care; they were skilled at masking the odors which penetrate even the most well-ventilated cancer room, and adept in the management of feeding with nasogastric, neck or abdominal wall intubation. These miserably time-consuming, emotionally stressful procedures (associated with massive local recurrence of cancer and the heroic attempts to control bleeding, drainage, odor, nutrition, respiration, pain and cosmesis) are, for the most part, things of the past. Our contemporary, more aggressive surgical or radiotherapeutic techniques serve to control local cancer in an ever-increasing number of patients. However, these patients more often die of metastatic disease and its associated complications of pulmonary insufficiency, hepatic dysfunction, renal failure and intestinal obstruction. Treatment may fail because of inability to control the dissemination of tumor cells and their implantation and growth in sites distant from the primary site. Thus, while aggressive therapy may cure an increasing number of patients, it may in some instances control only the local disease and, therefore, allow the patient to live long enough to develop the full manifestations of the disease. Metastases to distant sites, a phenomenon seldom noted in the past as a part of the head and neck cancer patient problem, is now unfortunately a much more prevalent problem than is local recurrence of tumor growth. Consideration must be given to the specifics of how to handle the urgent, or life-threatening or pain problems of the oral cancer patient just as it is given to caring for the patient whose primary cancer has developed in another site in the body.

Maintenance of Life

Cancer of the oral laryngeal-pharyngeal airway is most frequently a disease which develops in the person who has been a heavy consumer of alcohol. Nearly all of these patients are also excessive smokers. It is absolutely essential that the cured patient refrain from contact with these agents, but when it is apparent that cure can no longer be attained, satisfying the patient's drive for alcohol and tobacco may be more important than the worry of continued exposure to these carcinogenic agents.

Because metastic growth may be slow, the oral lesion which did not come to medical attention until it was incurable may exhibit local symptomatology for months before actual distress is experienced by the patient. It is this characteristic of tumor growth which requires patience and meticulous day-by-day management on the part of the attending staff. Much of the following discussion will be related primarily to the patient who is not in the actual terminal status of his tumor growth pattern. In contrast, the question of how heroic the procedures of day-to-day care should be in the case of the patient with large, exophytic oral cancer is another consideration altogether. The patient may be bedridden and relatively immobile; or he may be relatively active and held down only by the restriction of bleeding, odor and weakness due to nutritional deficiency. If there is a spontaneous massive hemorrhage, the question of heroic control is one the personal physician or nurse must decide. For the tumor that exhibits a bloody ooze or a necrotic discharge, pleasant relief often can be obtained by the use of frequent cauterizations and debridement. Some of the innovations in regional chemotherapy may offer temporary remission of tumor growth, but seldom does this result in what is interpreted as good terminal care management. The innovations in cryosurgery, whereby extremes of subfreezing temperatures are delivered to a tumor, can offer significant palliation in many of the oral lesions.

Cosmesis

Some significant degree of cosmetic disfigurement as a result of previous treatment is not unusual in the cancer-bearing patient. This may be due to severe contractural deformities and skin changes resulting from irradiation or surgical excision. These patients have often acclimated themselves to changes in their physical appearance and so find themselves not unusually distressed by the appearance of a large tumor growth showing on the face or neck.

Yet other patients and their families will not tolerate situations of extreme cosmetic deformity and may call upon the oncologist to perform the impossible. Palliative attempts at excising tumor masses are seldom worthwhile, further radiation is usually not advisable and thus the patient becomes separated from the familiar environmental surroundings which he so badly needs. Sedation, dressings which cover the tumor, and bed-immobilization or isolation may serve to protect the family but are not acceptable procedures unless the patient has lost awareness of his surroundings. There are no definitive answers to these problems of the management of the terminally ill. Each situation must be approached as a unique one and handled with concern for the needs of all the individuals involved.

Maintenance of Nutrition

The terminal patient may suffer from swallowing difficulties resulting from surgery or extreme dryness of the mouth resulting from radiation. When the growth of the cancer mass obstructs proper oral intake of food in the otherwise comfortable and relatively ambulatory patient, energetic attempts can be carried out, without undue morbidity, which will allow good nutritional maintenance. Attempts to maintain nutritional adequacy through the use of intravenous hyperalimentation techniques are not appropriate on a long-term basis. Similarly, the use of a nasal gastric or oral gastric inserted feeding tube is not a procedure which is convenient to the patient. Preferably, a small caliber tube should be inserted into the pharynx or cervical esophagus, thereby providing a means for maintaining nutrition. Cervical feeding tube esophagostomy is a procedure with which more clinicians should become familiar since it serves as a comfortable and convenient means of maintaining good nutrition.

(Seldom, if ever, is there a good clinical indication to add to the patient's morbidity by using a trans-abdominally placed gastrostomy tube. In general, it is poorly tolerated by most patients. The patient has to position himself accurately to use this tube for feeding and the site drains every time food material is placed into the stomach, making frequent dressing changes necessary.)

Significant improvement in nutritional maintenance can be obtained with the techniques described above even in the patient with a large head and neck tumor. The actual indications for their use, however, will often depend upon the judgment of the doctor in charge. It must be remembered that patients who have surgery or radiation to the oral, laryngeal or pharyngeal area seldom, if ever, have a normal sense of smell and taste. Cognizance must be given to the fact that one of the problems in maintaining nutrition in these patients is their actual lack of desire for food rather than their inability to eat.

Hygiene

Drooling. As a result of cancer treatment, or of tumor growth itself, the patient may have the distress of drooling. The approach to this problem in the patient who is free of local oral cancer may differ from the one utilized with the patient who has a large growing tumor. If there is no evidence of local recurrence of cancer, the drooling might be controlled by the use of anticholinergic agents or by minimal plastic reconstructive procedures which would deepen the buccal gutters or the floor of the mouth. It is helpful if the patient is encouraged to learn to swallow adequately and frequently. Yet learning to swallow with a physical intra-oral defect due either to anatomical dysfunction or tumor growth is as difficult as learning the use of esophageal speech after laryngectomy. Little reluctance should be experienced in proceeding with radiation to the salivary glands to depress salivary flow. Some success has also been obtained by ligation of the major salivary ducts.

Angular stomatitis and circumoral dermatitis due to the irritating components of oral fluids, as well as due to infection itself, may complicate the drooling problem and should be treated by topical applications of appropriate medications.

Odor. The odor from a necrotic tumor might not be any worse than the odor from a mouth exhibiting poor hygiene. The result is nonetheless distressing and proper procedures should be followed if the morale of the patient is to be maintained. Among the many problems worthy of discussion, none can be more important than that continued emphasis be placed on maintaining close family-patient, nurse-patient and physician-patient rapport, but this is difficult to do if the odor problem is not adequately controlled. Mouth irrigations alone will not take care of poor hygiene. The dentist must be asked to assist in teeth care and the management of inflammatory conditions of the gums. Use of the toothbrush, water pick and dental floss are all mandatory. Dental plaque on the intra-oral prosthesis, or on the teeth themselves, must be energetically controlled if the odor from both the tumor and the oral cavity is to be controlled. Adequate room ventilation, frequent tumor debridement by one of several means, the use of pleasant room deodorizers and frequent dressing and bed clothes changes are of great assistance.

Infection. Oral moniliasis occurs frequently in the cancer patient. This can be the result of general debilitation, malnutrition, therapy attempts such as irradiation or chemotherapeutic drugs and, of course, antibiotics, physio-pharmacological agents and corticosteroids. Aphthous stomatitis and other local infectious processes are best controlled by the good hygienic measures of tumor cleansing astringent mouth washes and, on occasion, use of antibiotic rinses.

Pain. Just as the patient who has undergone extensive head and neck surgery experiences little pain postoperatively, similarly the oral cancer patient has minimal pain problems from local tumor. The infected tooth or the blocked sinus are more often the cause of pain. However, the trismus that might result from pterygoid muscle infiltration with tumor can be uncomfortable, as can actual invasion of the bone by the tumor. More often the need for pain medication in the oral cancer patient is related to patient anxiety, discomfort and emotional distress, rather than true pain itself. (This has been repeatedly demonstrated by allowing the patient to return to his drinking habits and the use of tobacco, whether it be cigarette, cigar or snuff.) Most oncologists have come to the general agreement that when pain medication is needed, it should be administered rather aggressively.

We often observe the distress of the patient who has become addicted to narcotics over a long period of usage and whose pain now is one of addiction rather than the pain of actual tumor invasion. It is the author's experience that the pain of addiction is much more severe than any pain due to cancer invasion alone. Experienced judgment must be exercised before these patients are allowed to become addicted, as they eventually will be, no matter how much care and discretion might be used by the doctor and the nurse in the administering of narcotics. Some of the less-addicting agents have been helpful, but it has been shown that they, too, will have the same addicting-type of effect if used long enough. Every attempt should be made to hold off the addicting-type of medication until that time when the physician is emotionally ready to use it in rather large doses in an energetic way.

It should be remembered that the patient's pain may not be from the tumor directly but from secondary infection or irritating agents, such as food and liquids, or from the intra-oral dental prosthesis. The oral cancer patient is often prone to dental abnormalities such as caries, odontogenic infections, defective fillings and periodontal disease. The relief of these conditions may show that they were, essentially, the sole source of distressing pain. Therefore, the maintenance of good oral hygiene is one of the prime factors in the control of pain.

The use of peripheral nerve interruption, accomplished by alcohol or aqueous phenol injections, is occasionally of benefit. Cranial nerve sectioning as well as prefrontal leucotomy will change the patient's experience with pain. One sometimes wonders at the results of neuronectomy procedures and questions whether the pain-relief results primarily from the personality changes brought about by the operation. The removal of necrotic, exposed bone will frequently bring pain problems under control.

Summary

A lifetime of caring for the oral cancer patient, both those who have been cured and those for whom treatment has failed, in no way allows the author to answer all the questions related to the care of the terminal oral cancer patient. It must be remembered that the growth characteristics of each cancer are unique unto themselves; each cancer is unique in the way it affects individual patients; and each patient is unique in the manner in which he handles his problems related to terminal care. Seldom does the patient need misguided sympathy but he does need understanding and frankness about the problems he is facing and must face in the immediate future.

Oral Care of the Dying Patient
(With Special Reference to the Oral Cancer Patient)
S. Gordon Castigliano*

With the advent of cardiac transplantation, the definition of death has taken on a complexity scarcely imagined a few short years ago. The stethoscope and the palpating fingers are far from adequate proof of death by today's strict standards. If death itself is so difficult to determine to the satisfaction of all, almost certainly no one can satisfactorily define that point in time when a person has reached a dying state. At death one deals with the absolute. On the other hand, there is nothing that is fixed or irrevocable about the dying state.

For example, about seven decades ago, a famous surgeon after operating on one hundred consecutive breast cancer patients could not boast of having cured a single patient. They all died of the disease. Today, a patient with cancer of the breast enjoys quite a different and far more hopeful outlook. Seventy years ago those breast cancer patients in actuality were doomed from the outset based on the then existing knowledge. They were, in fact, dying patients. Today this would not be so.

Strictly speaking, death is a long process which begins at birth. Each passing day brings closer that day of final dissolution. The more knowledgeably and skillfully life is lived, the greater is the likelihood of protraction and delay of that fateful day. In this context, the oral care of a dying patient would be a lifelong process. If, however, the dying patient is to be regarded as one whose remaining life can be measured in weeks or months, remarks dealing with oral care can be considerably contracted.

Until all patients seek diagnosis and treatment while the neoplastic disease is in a curable stage, practicing physicians will be confronted with the difficult task of caring for the terminal cancer patient. It can be safely stated, on the basis of current data, that today nearly four out of five advanced cancer patients will go through the terminal stage and die. Thus, it is appropriate to intensify our efforts to promote the well-being of this large segment of our dying population. The care of the oral cavity constitutes an important aspect of the overall care of all dying patients.

It has been established that approximately 100 days represent the average remaining life span of the terminal cancer patient. Some will live

---

*Chief, Head and Neck Service, American Oncological Hospital, Philadelphia, Pennsylvania

months longer while some will survive just a few short weeks after being classified as terminal. The cancer patient nearly always prefers to spend his last days at home in familiar and friendly surroundings. This may not always be possible or even desirable. There may be firm indications for the patient to be hospitalized to meet or prevent certain impending complications. Although it is true that many terminal cancer patients require hospitalization, there is no evidence to show that such care extends the patient's life even though better care may be given. Basically, the best care for the terminal cancer patient is one which supports morale, promotes comfort, and strives to preserve the family's financial resources. These goals can often be best achieved at home. It must be recognized that many patients properly assessed as being in the dying stage are not yet to be classed as terminal. Such patients may require careful and well-executed therapy of some kind, be it surgery, irradiation or anti-tumor chemotherapy alone or in combination.

Any hospital facility which purports to treat the chronically ill, including the incurable and therefore dying cancer patient, must be at least as competent to treat the disease as a general hospital. Today, under Medicare and pressure from utilization committees, the patient's stay in the hospital is being shortened and his discharge to nursing homes, where in too many cases adequate care is not available, is hastened. Physicians generally are cooperating to avoid unjustified criticism and in some cases even impugnation and censure. We must come to grips with the fact that the chronically ill patient belongs in the same setting as the short-term patient, if good care is to be given him. High quality care must be made easier for patients to obtain—not more difficult. The dying patient with or without cancer is entitled to the *best* care. Quite obviously, some patients in the dying state can be adequately managed in well-operated and properly equipped and staffed nursing homes or in other cases even at home.

When home care is planned, the physician may draw from a number of willing untrained volunteers within the patient's family and spend some time training them. If necessary in special instances, private nursing maybe obtained and, in many instances, a practical nurse can perform adequately. A member of the Visiting Nurses Association can be contacted to call regularly, but careful doctor's orders must be left for the nurse. Occasionally, assistance in housekeeping and help in other basic ways can be obtained by contacting the local American Cancer Society.

Philosophy of Terminal Oral Care

In considering recommendations for the oral care of the dying patient, the patient's prospects for survival must be carefully assessed. An attempt at accurate assessment of the duration of life remaining for a patient is important in properly guiding those charged with oral care. For example, the removal of many teeth and subsequent prosthetic replacement may be indicated when relatively long time survival seems a strong likelihood. On the other hand, such an approach would be unwise in a patient whose life expectancy is measured in a few short months. There exist certain instances, however, in which the patient's complaints are strong and demanding and his morale needs a boost, so that exceptions can and must be made. Evaluation of all factors involved is essential. At no time should the decision damage the patient's morale, and the temptation to overmanage the patient's problem should be avoided. The long-term dying patient constitutes an expensive ordeal for everyone concerned. Adequate substitutes for costly oral care can be found and nearly always can satisfy the needs of the patient.

Oropharyngeal cancer patients may enter the dying stage after having received previous adequate or inadequate oral care. The elimination of sepsis, removal of unhealthy teeth, scaling of dental plaque, persistent use of fluoride and daily hygiene are the keys to this care. With a hopeless patient, however, there is less need for such strict oral care. The mouth should not be neglected, but common sense should be exercised. If the patient has little chance of surviving six months, few teeth should be removed unless strongly indicated.

Removal of teeth in a post-irradiated field even where megavoltage has been used is never to be regarded as a safe procedure. Every conservative effort should be made to save teeth. Only after conservative therapy fails and absolute indications exist should extraction be undertaken. The extraction should be done in as atraumatic a manner as possible. Ample pre- and post-extraction antibiotic coverage should be maintained.

The patient should report frequently to a dentist who is well informed in the management of post-irradiated teeth. If the personal dentist feels that he would prefer the patient to be cared for by the clinic or hospital dentist, this should be arranged. Another alternative is care shared among the therapist, hospital dentist, and personal dentist.

Strictly speaking, insofar as the patient with head and neck cancer is concerned, when the patient is no longer able to care for himself, he should be regarded as in need of special care. This time can be postponed by a variety of ways in the total care of the patient. The better the dying patient is cared for, the longer the patient will be willing, desirous, and able to care for his own oral needs. He will, of course, require special skills for special situations.

In summary, only oral procedures deemed to be essential within the period of life expectancy should be performed. It is usually of little value to subject patients who are doomed to die in a short time to involved and expensive dental care.

Specific Dental and Oral Care

The dentulous and edentulous terminal care patient should be maintained in an oral environment as nearly optimum as possible without violating basic common sense tenets. Generally, the edentulous patient poses fewer problems. The hygienic oral care of the terminal patient should be under the management of a dentist trained in the care of such cases.

Teeth should be cleaned and scaled at regular and frequent intervals and the mouth generally maintained in as good condition as practicable. This is not always easy to accomplish and may call for the assistance of personnel of other specialities. The patient's mouth should be corrected of gross sepsis. In addition, snags of teeth should be removed. Further, the patient should be taught the essential rudiments of home care. These would be, for example:

1) the proper approach to oral hygiene, including the proper type of toothbrush to use and its correct method of use;
2) how to set up and use oral irrigating equipment;
3) how to recognize dental plaque with the use of disclosing agents and how to remove the plaque;
4) how to use fluoride gels and fluoride carriers properly;
5) the avoidance of physical, thermal, and chemical trauma to prevent possible osteonecrosis; (ill-fitting dentures or obturators should be modified when indicated; strenuous use of dentures should be avoided; prostheses should be worn only when essential, to avoid the undue trauma of continual use; overuse of irritating topical anesthesia should be avoided);
6) the importance and need of frequent periodic check-ups.

A strict program of oral care reduces the incidence of serious complications and brings the dying patient to the terminal stage of his disease with the oral cavity in a condition able to endure the final days in relative comfort.

Hairy and heavily coated tongue should be adequately cared for. The heavily coated furry tongue often contributes directly to the dying patient's general distress. Currettement of the tongue in the patient who is tube fed or eating a non-detergent liquid or soft type dietary is frequently necessary. The instruments which have been found to be most useful are a large cervical currette, a bent teaspoon, or a fixed looped corset stave.

At all times we must strive to accomplish our objective without unnecessary depletion of the family finances. It seems useless to subject a patient to needless discomfort and expense when death is so near. This is not to say that carious teeth causing distress should not be attended to. Occasionally an absolute indication will develop for the removal of a tooth. However, this must never be done without consultation with the oncologist, surgeon or therapist in charge. If tooth extraction is agreed upon, adequate pre-extraction antibiotic coverage as well as protracted antibiotic coverage following extraction are necessary. It must be emphasized that extraction of teeth from irradiated bone must never be regarded as a safe procedure. A fulminating acute osteonecrosis may be set in motion.

In cases of dental breakdown following irradiation the use of fluoride internally and locally can do much to delay or forestall the need for extraction. In other cases, the careful use of heavy applications of 20 per cent silver nitrate to the disintegrating crowns of teeth will slow down disintegration to the point where removal will not be needed. This procedure must be performed by one experienced in its use. In cases with fractured crowns where the above treatment does not control the situation, crown amputation to the gingival level can be done. Root fillings can be carried out to delay extraction. Every attempt should be made to save the teeth. Even in the case of apical abscess, drainage without extraction should be attempted first.

Irradiation Osteonecrosis

The oral cancer patient suffering from uncontrolled or recurrent disease following irradiation therapy delivered in the near or distant past needs carefully supervised oral care. Such a patient may or may not have osteonecrosis. The osteonecrosis may be localized or may be extensive. There may be fracture or fracture may be imminent. The philosophy of management of osteonecrosis in the dying patient varies depending on the length of time the patient is expected to live. Patients treated by orthovoltage irradiation will often require a different approach to management from those cases treated by megavoltage irradiation. Patients treated by megavoltage (supervoltage-teleocobalt, etc.) can often be treated conservatively. In any case when the patient's prospects for survival are poor, no surgical procedures should be contemplated other than possible rongeuring and moulding sharp fragments. Activated zinc peroxide packing is helpful in the area of exposed and breaking down bone. (See Odor and Infection for further details of management.) If many months of survival seem likely in cases where large and painful exposure of the mandible is present, more extensive procedures, such as large sequestrectomies and even intra-oral mandiblectomies, may be considered. In some cases of osteonecrosis, mandiblectomy may not be indicated, but the occasional patient suffering from severe and intolerable pain does require relief first.

Management of Pain

If pain is not controllable without resorting to opiates in high doses, the procedure of alcohol injection of the branches of the trigeminal nerve at the foramen ovale should be given strong consideration. Alcohol injection is also useful in non-osteonecrotic cases where the uncontrolled cancer produces unbearable pain. Peripheral injection is of no value. In some cases, injection of the gasserian ganglion itself is indicated, using the anterior approach through the foramen ovale after the method of Patrick and Dorrance. If the pain is pharyngeal as well as oral, injection of the fifth cranial nerve will prove inadequate. When the prospects for survival and severe suffering can be expected to be protracted for many months, craniotomy and section of pharyngeal nerve and upper cervical roots are worth considering.

Many oral cancer patients can receive adequate pain relief with ordinary medication. At first, only the mildest drugs should be used. In considering the mild drugs such as aspirin, it should be remembered that a good night's sleep is important preparation for bearing the rigors of living or dying another day. Sleep can be promoted with a variety of available medications. Tranquilizers, likewise, should be used early, along with mood elevators. Nor should alcohol be forgotten. A tendency exists among some physicians to prescribe opiates in soporific diurnal doses early in the terminal stage of oral cancer. Such treatment not only is unneeded, it is unwarranted. Only the smallest doses of narcotic to produce the desired effect should be prescribed. It must be emphasized, however, that the patient should not be allowed to suffer. Darvon, Talwin, Codeine and Percodan may be used early. Topical anesthesia such as Xylocaine Viscous and Xylocaine Ointment impregnated in gauze, Benzocaine lozenges and paste, Nupercainal lozenges and Pontocaine (1% or 2%) spray can also be employed.

Frequent mouth washes with ordinary isotonic salt solution, with baking soda or some form of antacid give unbelievable relief. This should be done as often as every 15 minutes. Hydrogen peroxide solution in varying strengths (usually half strength) is cleansing and promotes comfort.

As seems indicated, one may proceed to Demerol, Dilaudid, Pantopon, and Morphine. Morphine in combination with Hyoscine and Caffeine may be necessary in the final stages. Intravenous alcohol can also be tried. Psychotherapy and hypnosis are worthy of occasional consideration. In rare cases, where pain cannot be relieved by other means, precision prefrontal lobotomy may be useful. Although the pain persists, the patient is no longer distressed by it. This procedure is to be reserved for unrelieved pain in low threshold patients suffering also from severe anxiety and emotional maladjustment.

Odor

Perhaps the most distressing feature in the history of some oral cancer patients is the foul putrid odor generated by the necrotic uncontrolled tumor and osteonecrotic irradiated bone. The family and the attendants are all distressed by the characteristic odor of sloughing malodorous breakdown products. The patient, to a large degree, is spared the odor. The oropharyngeal cancer patient treated by irradiation has usually some degree of anosmia and becomes tolerant or unaware of the odor.

The problem of odor has not been adequately controlled by methods currently available. Frequent dressing changes and irrigations with hydrogen peroxide and irrigations with weak solutions of Dakin's or Clorpactic solution are helpful. In general, the usual anti-infective mouth washes have little value. In some cases, surgical debridement may be absolutely necessary to remove odor sufficiently to permit nursing care of the patient. This procedure is not to be considered if the remaining days of life are few.

Aerosol sprays and methylsalicylate wicks are to be used within the room. Deodorizers operated by fans blowing air over cylinders of evaporable jellied counteractant deodorants are available.* Also available are air sprays for surface disinfection on door handles, light switches, bed springs, wheelchairs, waste cans, toilet facilities, dressing carts, spills and evacuations. Granular deodorizers are of value in some cases for use on floors, carpets, and waste receptacles used for vomit and excrements.

It should be mentioned that local or topical antibiotics seldom contribute importantly to the control of odor or infection in the necrotic tissues. However, Varidase may be helpful.

Infection

Oral moniliasis frequently complicates the terminal days of the dying patient and adds considerably to his discomfort. Moniliasis results from a combination of factors in the debilitated malnourished patient, who is, perhaps, suffering from chronic alcoholism and, generally, from the late effects of intensive unsuccessful irradiation. Moniliasis also finds fertile soil in patients overtreated with cancer chemotherapy, intensive antibiotic drugs and corticosteroids. A conclusive diagnosis can and should be made by means of cultures. Treatment consists of mouth rinses (four or more times a day) employing Mycostatin suspension. Applications of Mycostatin Ointment can also be used. Mycostatin oral tablets can be tried. Gentian violet is not worthwhile in the author's opinion and is most troublesome as it stains clothing and bedclothes.

The necessity for systemic treatment of infection in patients suffering with oral cancer generally results from continuing radiation osteonecrosis, breakdown and infection following palliative irradiation. Infection associated with leukopenia secondary to intensive anti-tumor chemotherapy or extensive irradiation, pneumonia due to debilitation aspiration, and stasis due to prolonged recumbency will also require systemic antibiotic therapy. The treatment consists of the elimination as far as is possible of underlying factors and the administration of systemic antibiotic therapy. (Food aspiration will require bronchoscopic suctioning in some cases.) The specific drug treatment should be selected after culture and sensitivity tests have indicated the nature of the infecting organism and the appropriate antibiotic agent.

---

* Osmefar (produced by Airkem Division of Airwick Industries, Inc.)

Xerostomia

Dryness of the mouth is a common complication resulting from the intensive irradiation therapy of the oral carcinoma. Xerostomia is particularly severe when the major salivary glands have been subjected to such therapy. There seems to be virtually no capacity for regeneration of the salivary glands after damage by irradiation. No satisfactory method is known whereby the atrophic salivary epithelium can be stimulated to produce saliva at levels which can be considered functional.

Xerostomia, with its symptoms of dryness, soreness, and general oral discomfiture is aggravated by alcohol, spicy foods, bulky dry foods, thermically hot foods, carbonated beverages and tobacco. In severe cases, the xerostomia may precipitate surface gingival erosions leading to distressing bone exposure and osteonecrosis. Although no invariably successful method of management for mouth dryness exists, a general approach to its management is worth discussing.

General body dehydration should be prevented by maintaining a proper fluid intake. An environment calculated to promote a dry mouth and nose should be avoided. The bedroom and living area of the home or hospital room should maintain a proper level of humidity. In a home where warm air heat is used, humidifiers should be employed. The air temperature should not be above 70°F, preferably 68°. When humidifiers are unavailable, flat pans of water should be placed near heat sources. Excessive use of automobile heaters should be avoided. Cool vaporizers should be used and may prove most helpful. Frequent mouth rinsing (with isotonic salt solution and baking soda); the application of vaseline to the lips, and mineral oil or glycerine with lemon juice to the oral mucous membranes assist in combating dryness. Lemon and glycerine swabs (a 50 per cent lemon juice and 50 per cent glycerine mixture) are available as a prepared and packaged product.* In the author's opinion, these swabs along with frequent oral irrigations and lavage are basic for the oral care in the dying patient.

Slippery elm cough drops, chewing gum (sugar-free), lemon drops, and cold water are useful adjuncts. Saturated solution of potassium iodide taken orally in increasing dosage, starting at doses of 5 drops t.i.d., increasing by one drop a day to doses of about XXX drops t.i.d., may stimulate salivary flow somewhat.

---

* Manufactured by Ipco Hospital Supply Company.

Patients with xerostomia suffer from tenacious mucous in mouth, throat, and bronchi. Many dying patients afflicted with dry mouth and throat also suffer varying degrees of emphysema and bronchitis and some may develop aspiration pneumonitis which may prove to be terminal. The use of Alevaire wets, dilutes, and loosens viscid respiratory secretions. It is made up of tyloxapol with sodium bicarbonate and glycerine. Alevaire should be administered full strength in a fine mist by an aerosol nebulizer. It may be used 30 to 90 minutes three times a day or constantly until relief is obtained (1 - 3 days). The nebulizer works off the regulator flow meter of an oxygen tank or connected to a suitable motor-driven air compressor. Mucomyst, 20 per cent, also can be used effectively. (A 10 per cent solution provides added convenience for home use in hand nebulizing units.)

Isuprel may be of value in cases where the amount of bronchial mucous should be reduced in an effort to promote comfort. In addition to diminishing mucous secretions, Isuprel reduces bronchial spasm and shrinks swollen mucous membranes. Isuprel is administered by oxygen aerosolization or by a hand nebulizer. Directions included with the medication should be followed carefully. Dosage should be adjusted for patients with complicating hyperthyroidism, limited cardiac reserve, coronary disease or specific allergy.

In patients with tracheostomy stomas, introduction of several cc of isotonic salt solution and weak sodium bicarbonate solution is helpful for loosening tenacious mucous. Proper, frequent and deep aspiration is never to be neglected and its use may be required more frequently following the use of mucolytic agents.

Ozena with nasal dryness, heavy crusting and odor may complicate intensive irradiation. Considerable relief is said to be obtained by daily irrigation with Karo syrup.

Oral Irrigation

Oral irrigation serves sveral purposes. It cleanses and removes odor soothes, and moistens the dry mucous membranes, thereby promoting a lift in morale. A salt and soda solution is commonly employed. This can be made by mixing one teaspoonful of table salt and one teaspoonful of baking soda with 1000 cc of warm water. As a substitute, a mixture of one ounce of milk of magnesia to 1000 cc of water is used occasionally. Another substitute is a mixture of one-half ounce of AlCaroid and 1000 cc of warm water. Less frequently used is one ounce of Maalox in 1000 cc of warm water. Hydrogen peroxide serves chiefly as a cleanser and can be used effectively following oral feedings. It can also be used half-strength in cases where a painful mucositis is present during and following palliative irradiation. In other cases, the conventional drug store 3 per cent concentration can be used.

The mechanics involved in oral irrigation vary. The solution may be mixed in a cup, taken into the mouth and swished and agitated to the best of the patient's ability. If this is too painful or the patient is physically unable to agitate and cleanse his mouth, other methods should be employed.

For example, a disposable enema unit can be employed for oral lavage.* This technique consists of flowing about one-half to one quart of any of the above described solutions in such a fashion as to cleanse the entire oral cavity. The end of the tubing should be fitted with a suitable nozzle or tip applicator with an aperture or orifice of about 1.5 to 2.5 mm. The procedure is performed under mild pressure which can be controlled by the degree of elevation of the container. Generally, a height of three to five feet above a sink or bowl is adequate. The solution should be comfortably warm. If the patient suffers from xerostomia, cold solutions may follow the preliminary lavage and will give the dry mouth longer-lasting comfort. The solution passes in and out of the mouth into a basin or a sink. The solution should be comfortably tolerated. Jet pressure devises are available and may be quite satisfactory in some cases after the acute phase of the mucositis is over, but the pressure must be controlled.**

Terminal cancer patients with a few short months to live who have received intensive, unsuccessful irradiation therapy require the same careful oral care as was prescribed and carried out earlier. The new status of "terminal cancer patient" does not mean that the mouth should be neglected. The rampant caries which follow intensive irradiation in the neglected dying patient are largely due to xerostomia. This should be prevented by continuing the strict regimen carried out earlier when the prospects for cure or long-term survival still existed.

This patient will have increased xerostomia, leading to plaque formation about the cervical areas of the teeth which will go on to produce rapid and destructive caries even outside the irradiated fields. The teeth

---

* Traversal Laboratories
** One such apparatus is the Water pic.

and gums should be cleaned regularly with soft multi-tufted toothbrushes. The ends of the filaments of the brush should be rounded to avoid trauma to the gingivae. In some near-terminal patients, a marked degree of trismus exists which makes oral care virtually impossible. This should be treated by dilators of which there are a variety of types. In some cases, relief of the trismus under short acting anesthesia is justifiable to make possible proper oral care. It should be mentioned again that fibrous trismus is best treated by prevention.

Plaque formation around the necks of the teeth should be removed regularly. This is best done by the dentist at frequent intervals, although the relatively alert and ambulatory patient can carry out an adequate removal of plaque. Dental plaque removal is basically important in the preservation of the integrity of irradiated and non-irradiated teeth in the patient suffering from xerostomia. This aspect of oral care must not be abandoned and can be aided by the use of disclosing agents.

As the patient's condition worsens, dehydration becomes an added factor and mouth breathing and fistula formation further dry the mucous membranes. The tongue becomes heavily furred and the mucous membranes parched and sore. Such a tongue and mouth do much to promote the patient's feeling of deep malaise and impending death. A clean mouth or as clean a mouth as possible does much to elevate the spirits. When the patient notes that dentists and other paramedical attendants are interested in maintaining oral hygiene and request his cooperation, his spirits are given a real boost. A clean, moist mouth with a good taste does much to brighten the spirits and gives strength to endure the rigors of those final days.

The importance of a clean mouth to the dying patient still has not sufficiently impressed the average physician or nurse. In the author's experience the care of the dying patient's mouth is a sorely neglected facet of his overall care.

Drooling

Excessive salivation or inability to swallow saliva may cause drooling. This problem may become quite distressing to the patient. Control of drooling is a difficult problem and is seldom successfully accomplished. Ingenious suction devices sometimes can be contrived. A small mushroom catheter placed in the floor of the mouth exiting through a tight opening in the submaxillary area can be utilized in troublesome cases. Generally, reassurance and training the patient to swallow differently and more frequently may help. Anticholinergic agents such as Belladonna derivatives, Pro-Banthine, etc., and tranquilizers possessing antisialagogue activity can be tried. In severe cases after surgical management, irradiation therapy to the major salivary glands is worthy of a trial.

In dying patients whose survival time is deemed to be limited, simple ligation of major salivary ducts deserves consideration when drooling causes severe angular eczematoid dermatitis and general distress. The dermatitis results from the constant irritating moisture on the skin and infecting organisms from the oral flora. Conservative treatment consists of the use of waterproof grease (obtained from a plumber's shop) or aluminum paste. Mycolog ointment can be used in the presence of infection with C. albicans. When secondary infection from staph or strep is present, the above treatment can be alternated with Neo-Cortef cream. Severe cases of eczematoid dermatitis arising from sensitivity to the patient's own discharges can be treated with local compresses of one-quarter of one per cent silver nitrate solution for 30 minutes three or four times a day. Silicones may be tried.* Occasionally, corticosteroid creams may provide remarkable relief.

Carotid Body Syndrome

When metastatic disease grows uncontrolled in the neck or shrinks, contracts and becomes rigid and deeply fixed following radiotherapy, abnormal pressure is produced against the carotid sinus which affects the pulse and blood pressure. Undue pressure may cause fatal syncope. Patients with large fixed cervical masses should be cautioned about turning the head from side to side as this may trigger an attack of syncope.

Treatment consists of maintaining an open respiratory tract passageway and the use of atropine sulfate by subcutaneous injection. Paredrine hydrobromide can be used as a preventive, 20 to 60 mg daily.

Hemorrhage

Severe bleeding often occurs in uncontrolled intra-oral malignant neoplastic disease. Local packing or attempts at local intra-oral ligation is almost never of any value. The bleeding results from erosion of the blood vessel wall by invasive tumor and local measures cannot be expected to control the problem. There is perhaps no more alarming catastrophe for

---

* Covicone cream (Abbott) and Silicote Skin Protective Spray or Cream (Arnar-Stone).

the patient than severe intra-oral bleeding and prompt decisive action should be taken. Temporary packing even with digital pressure may prove necessary while arranging for and during ligation of the external carotid artery and branches on the bleeding side and occasionally on the contralateral side as well. Occasionally, due to extensive metastatic disease, common carotid artery ligation on the affected side may be the only feasible procedure with possible contralateral lingual artery ligation. This procedure carries a danger of paralysis, or death may occur.

Nutrition and the Oral Cavity

Mastication and swallowing in many cases become increasingly difficult and not infrequently impossible. Gastrostomy in such cases is almost never indicated. A patient unable to swallow is fed by tube. Generally, a No. 16 or 18 caliber naso-gastric tube suffices. Occasionally, the patient tolerates the naso-gastric tube poorly. In such cases a naso-gastric tube of soft penrose drain rubber can be made. The least troublesome long-term feeding tube technique is that of placing an ordinary No. 16 or 18 tube in the low lateral pharynx or cervical esophagus by means of a relatively simple operative procedure. Care must be taken to avoid placement of the terminal end of the feeding tube in the duodenum. This causes a dumping syndrome. The patient occasionally can use an ordinary urinary catheter and place the tube prior to a feeding and on completion remove the tube himself.

The patient's diet can be quite simple. Although food supplements such as hydrolized proteins are often desirable, generally most food and liquids prepared for family table use can be adequately liquified with food blenders and swallowed by the patient. Formulas for tube feeding are readily available. In extreme cases, parenteral mixtures can be used.

Repeated aspiration of food and saliva into the trachea and bronchial tree may lead to intermittent attacks of aspiration pneumonia which can result in a terminal necrotizing pneumonia. Salivary and food aspiration follows operative procedures when both superior laryngeal nerves are cut in resecting the tumor. Bronchial aspiration may also follow operations where the epiglottis is totally removed with the tongue. In such cases, it may be of value to split the cricopharyngeus muscle.

When patients are able to masticate and swallow, the mouth should be irrigated following each intake of food. The patients should be encouraged to chew and swallow as long as possible. Foods skillfully and colorfully prepared are more appealing to the weakened patient. Mood elevators and alcohol can play an important role in giving the patient a much needed psychological lift and improved appetite.

Terminal or near terminal patients are frequently on concentrated low bulk, low residue diets. They will often complain of constipation. Fecal impaction occurs and should be thought of, looked for, and corrected. Constipation is an individual problem. Frequently of value in the management of this type of constipation are the following: milk of magnesia, alone or combined with mineral oil, Maltsupex (Borcherdt), and Metamucil (Searle). Also useful are Kondremul (Smith, Miller, and Patch) and Surfak capsules (Floyd Bros.).

Smoking, Alcohol, and Oral Care

Some patients treated for mouth cancer continue to smoke. If these patients are smoking when they reach the dying stage of the disease, no useful purpose will be served by completely interdicting the use of tobacco. Smoking does increase the difficulties in oral care, but some patients seem to have a strong psychological need to continue smoking. The emotional trauma produced by the discontinuance of smoking in certain rigid patients may outweigh the possible gains. However, when the terminal patient is bedridden, he should not be permitted to smoke unless under close surveillance.

Alcohol can prove of value if judiciously employed in the terminal cancer patient. It can be administered orally or by means of intravenous infusion or both.

Death Precipitated by Treatment of Serious or Terminal Disease

The use of a variety of medicaments may prove necessary or may be worth trying to forestall death or reduce distress during the dying process. Some drugs, even those generally regarded to be harmless, may actually hasten death if not employed with consummate skill.

Oxygen therapy can be listed among the treatments that have become almost routine in the management of desperately sick oral cancer patients. Oxygen therapy is usually helpful and comforting. However, if high concentrations are given over protracted periods of time, harm can occur. In some instances, injudicious use of oxygen may determine and hasten the outcome.

A host of other complications may follow injudicious treatment of the dying patient and may hasten death. For example, acidosis may result from over-employment of isotonic saline solution. Frequent mercurial diuresis may produce thiamine deficiency which can lead to terminal heart block. Respiratory depression may follow over-usage of opiates. Gastrointestinal lesions may be precipitated by steroids. Lethal reactions can follow 5 FU therapy and other anti-tumor agents. Multiple complications may by induced by antibiotic therapy.

Anti-depressants which are monoamine-oxidase inhibitors such as Parnate, Marplan, Nardil, and Niamid are dangerous when combined with sedatives, narcotics, hypnotics, analgesics, muscle relaxants, sympathicomimetic drugs and alcohol. Therefore, as a general safety rule monoamine-oxidase inhibitors should not be used in the dying oral cancer patient, unless under the supervision of a physician widely experienced in their use(1).

The Dentist's Role in Oral Care of the Dying Patient

The practicing dentist may wonder why he should be asked to interest himself in the dying patient. He has been asked to devote his energies to the preservation of teeth, their removal when preservation no longer is possible or advisable, and replacement in a variety of ingenious ways. More recently, he has been asked to contribute to the solution of the problem of early diagnosis in mouth cancer and also to participate in treating the various dental aspects of mouth cancer.

It seems appropriate to suggest that the dentist could perform a useful role in the care of the mouth in the case of the terminal or potentially terminal patient faced with death from any cause. All dying patients deserve the expert care that can be given them by one skilled in the treatment of oral disease related to the teeth. Outcome of any given critical illness is not predictable with certainty, and professional oral care may contribute importantly to a patient's comfort.

Classification of Dying Patients

Those responsible for the oral care of the dying patient must avoid the strong temptation to overemphasize the magnitude of their task. The dentist should refrain from doing more than is required or necessary for the projected life span of the patient. An accurate assessment of survival time should be made. In other words, is the patient curable or incurable? If incurable, are the prospects for survival measured in months or weeks? Survival studies of untreated and treated patients suffering from oral malignancy have been made. The average untreated oral cancer patient will be dead a short 18 months after the diagnosis, which is made an average of four months after the first symptom. After unsuccessful therapy, survival time is less than one year, on the average. The average terminal stage is about one hundred days.

After the patient is first seen and clinically investigated and categorized, he will be a candidate for either of two basic forms of management. First, he may be a candidate for attempts at curative surgery or irradiation therapy or a combination of both. Second, he may be a candidate for purely palliative treatment: surgical, irradiation, chemotherapy.* The patient who is earmarked for palliation may be regarded as a dying patient. Whatever palliative or ancillary oral therapy is planned for him should be considered in the pure light of this fact. The patient must not be overmanaged, nor must he be neglected. Neglect may drive him to seek help from a quack.

Palliative therapy (with megavoltage or supervoltage and/or Cobalt 60 irradiation) implies conservative therapy. Conservative treatment should not be interpreted to mean indifferent treatment. Patients with far-advanced cancer are as deserving of carefully executed therapy as the earlier cases. It is well known that in exceptional cases of far-advanced disease where the balance in growth rate, host resistance to disease and radio-responsiveness are optimum, inexplicably long-term survivals tantamount to cure may be experienced.

However, it must be stated here that the radiation therapist who sets out in an unrestrained effort to destroy every hopeless oral cancer that comes his way will fail to perform his task as a physician. He will not prolong life, nor will he alleviate suffering; rather, he may hasten death and, what is perhaps worse, he may add immeasurably to the patient's great discomfort. The same applies to the chemotherapist.

There is evidence to indicate that some cases of hopeless oral cancers are overtreated by surgery, irradiation therapy, or anti-tumor chemotherapy. It must be borne in mind that every cancer death after wild and futile surgery or overtreatment with irradiation or various chemotherapeutic anti-cancer agents adds to the army of dismal propagandists who believe that cancer is veritably incurable or who believe that surgery and/or heavy treatment not only shortens life by speeding the progress of the disease but actually makes the disease less bearable. Every oral cancer patient in the hopelessly advanced state who dies after ill-conceived radical surgery will leave behind a family physician, a family

*Chorio-epithelioma in some instances may be cured by chemotherapy.

dentist, mother, father, brothers, sisters and friends, many of whom will spread the gospel of despair.

It is probable, indeed likely, that many cancer deaths of today could be traced to the defeatist and apathetic attitude which led to a delay in treatment. Patients have developed fears directly as a result of disastrous or unhappy results in those who have been unwisely selected for operation. Operating on the inoperable is not a new pastime. What is new is that capable and vocal men are caught up in doing extensive palliative surgical exercise on hopeless cancer patients. It must be emphasized that radical surgery should be reserved for those patients in whom the prospects for cure are brightest.

Preservation of dignity in the dying patient is ignored too often. At no time in life is this more important. The proper focus of clinical medicine should be the *total* care and *total* regard for the welfare of the patient rather than the selfish scientific interest in the disease.

As has been pointed out by Dr. Walter Alvarez ". . . one of the essential qualities of the clinician is interest in humanity, for the secret of the care of the patient is in caring for the patient" (2).

Is Active Therapy Justifiable in the Dying Patient?

Active therapy by means of irradiation or anti-tumor chemotherapeutic agents is justifiable and may prove worthwhile. The treatment has limited objectives and this fact should never be forgotten. When previously untreated cervical metastatic disease is advancing rapidly, treatment will do much to boost patient morale by exerting growth restraint on the tumor. When irradiation therapy is no longer a method of choice, anti-tumor chemotherapeutic agents can be used with some beneficial effect. Rarely, infusion and perfusion techniques may be worthwhile.

It is fitting here to quote F. J. Ayd :

"Only when there is reasonable hope of sustaining life for several weeks or months, and if during this time the patient can be made comfortable should we exert every effort to delay death. Otherwise life-preserving treatment ceases to be a gift and becomes instead a scientific weapon for the prolongation of agony.

"As physicians we must recognize the dignity of man and his right to live and to die peacefully. If we do not do so, we are failing to strike a balance between the science and the art of medicine, to the detriment of our profession and the degradation of our fellow men—our patients" (3).

Yes, active therapy is justifiable in the dying patient, but let the following thought be remembered well! The inviolability of the dignity of the dying must come to be recognized as an inalienable and nontransferrable personal right, not to be breached or usurped even by the attending physician.

Voluntary Euthanasia

Because of the recent increase in discussion on the subject of euthanasia, a few remarks may be appropriate.

A sharp distinction must be made between the terms "voluntary euthanasia" and "ordinary euthanasia" or so-called mercy killing. There are advocates of both. In voluntary euthanasia, the patient asserts a moral right to decide for himself when his life should come to an end. A recent volume, *Euthanasia and the Right to Death* by A. B. Downing (4), presents 11 perceptive essays by eminent authorities in different fields. These advocates of legalizing voluntary euthanasia dissociate themselves from those who would support the right of the state to take the life of the senile, the mentally defective, or the incurable. They do, however, try to make a case for voluntary euthanasia. These authors contend that each person should have the freedom to choose between "a dignified and a squalid death."

In spite of the reasoning behind such views, there seems to be little difference between voluntary euthanasia and mercy killing. In either case, the physician's judgment is involved, since it is he who must "decide" that the patient is incurable. To legalize euthanasia in any form would place terrible responsibility in the hands of the physician and equally terrible doubts in the mind of the patient.

The Final Days

The final days for the oral cancer patient are difficult to bear. Everything possible should be done to support his morale. Mood elevators of various kinds should be tried. Corticosteroids can help. The physician and paramedical aides must be especially attentive to the patient. Professional neglect stems from a feeling of professional futility; this negativism communicates. The patient wants to see his doctor in whom he has faith and from whom he draws emotional sustenance.

Psychological Care of the Oral Cancer Patient

The patient with cancer in any site should associate himself with the possible challenge of death. This association with new concepts and attitudes requires assistance. The source for this help will rarely come from the physician who himself is generally uninformed about this facet of a patient's needs. Mental preparation for possible, impending or imminent death is certainly not a simple matter and calls for assistance from disciplines not generally found in the background and training of the cancer surgeon or irradiation therapist. The theologian, psychologist or psychiatrist may make a contribution. It seems likely that the people best suited for this task will be the pastoral counselors—men of all faiths who are graduates of seminaries, with at least three years of practice as clergymen and special post-graduate training in this kind of work. The graduate training ordinarily involves at least two years of internship and is served in hospitals.

Quite obviously, the patient's personal pastor plays a key part but often he himself will recognize the need for help. This is where the pastoral counselor comes in as a full-time specialist and consultant.

The oral cancer patient properly counseled and buttressed with knowledge can face death and endure the act of dying with courage and dignity. But he needs help—help from his cancer surgeon or irradiation therapist or both, from his family physician and dentist, from his pastor and family, and from the nurse, and every other employee of the hospital.

For the Future

Despite the continuing advance of bio-medical knowledge, death can not be denied—merely delayed.

All people now living have a common destiny—death—and all will require terminal care, save those few who will die suddenly of some catastrophe.

To improve the present generally unsatisfactory terminal care, it seems imperative that an ever-increasing effort be brought to bear in advancing the physical, emotional and spiritual amelioration of our final days.

Let those in policymaking positions strive to place the custody of our final days in the control of those whose supreme concern is the patient rather than the callous and self-serving search for knowledge of transient and even dubious value. Knowledge must not be gained at the expense of our dying. The price is too high. The gain is too little.

Bibliography

"Maintenance of Oral and General Health in the Management of the Oral Cancer Patient," American Cancer Society, Inc., 1968, 1969.

"Oral Care for Oral Cancer Patients," Washington, D. C.: U. S. Department of Health, Education, and Welfare, Public Health Service Publication.

References

1. "Death Owing to Treatment in Seriously Ill Patients." *Medical Science,* April 1967, p. 37.
2. W. Alvarez, Editorial. *Modern Medicine,* October 5, 1970, p. 100.
3. F. J. Ayd, *Journal of the American Medical Association, 181*:13, September 29, 1962.
4. A. B. Downing, *Euthanasia and the Right to Death. New York: Humanities Press, 1970.*

Hermes and Beyond†

*Ian W. D. Henderson**

In this the latter part of the twentieth century, the role of the physician has changed in regard to both its social context and its therapeutic goals. There is presently at the disposal of all physicians not only the considerable knowledge of disease prevention on a grand scale, but for those diseases which are not yet of negligible incidence, medication capable of cure or masking of the dysfunction by replacement, or at the worst, of amelioration of symptoms. Surgery and anesthesia have advanced to the point where every organ is now accessible to treatment, and replacement procedures are well established in a technical sense. Thus the relative number of patients who can look forward to cure and the return to a normal life has increased from the small percentage that existed one or two medical generations ago to the majority of those who seek our aid. With the powerful tools of modern pharmacology and the extraordinary surgical skills at our disposal, who can blame our space age patients from expecting to be cured even in the face of extremely serious illnesses —even cancer? No longer is the image of a physician as Hermes with his Caduceus escorting the dead across the river Styx into Hades acceptable; rather we are to escort those who are venturing too close to the river bank to safer ground.

Personnel who work daily in the field of malignant disease are faced constantly with decisions that may result in cure, but may at the same time mutilate and change the entire pattern of a patient's life. This is particularly true in cancer surgery and is perhaps more noticeable when the external appearance presented to the world is radically changed by a surgical intervention. It is in these cases that we must ponder the ethics of treatment of cancers of the palate, the tongue, floor of the mouth, gingiva, lips, the nasal sinuses and the upper respiratory tract. Despite the

---

† Although this chapter speaks mainly of the physician's role in the psychosocial care of the dying patient, its message is addressed to all other members of the health team. Indeed, everyone involved in the oral care of the terminal patient should consider his role as being parallel—psychosocially—to that of the physician.

* Department of Pharmacology, Faculty of Medicine, University of Ottawa, Ontario, Canada

availability of prosthetic devices which can be introduced to cover a large defect of the palate, a return to normal life is difficult for these patients; for those who require a glossectomy or a hemi-mandibulectomy, and suffer permanent disfigurement as well as difficulty in talking and eating, a return to normality is well-nigh impossible. This is true also for the unfortunate patient who must lose his larynx so that normal speech is forever lost, although many manage to communicate by a means of esophageal belching.

Radiation therapy given for malignant diseases of the oral cavity and the nasopharynx leaves the patient in an equally unenviable situation. Saliva is permanently decreased and any teeth that have remained in the mouth usually become carious at a time when removal may not be feasible. Equally dreaded is the complication of radiation necrosis of bone which produces pain of such severity that patients quickly become addicted to narcotics. Cancer chemotherapy, too, produces deleterious effects within the oral cavity, for the cells of that area are unusually sensitive to many of the anti-metabolic agents. Last but not least, the oral cavity is often the site of "opportunistic" infections such as Candidiasis, or even the more dreadful Mucormycosis that starts in the nasopharynx and may then spread to the brain and the orbit.

Although definitive treatment by surgery, radiation therapy and chemotherapy can cure a significant number of patients, an even larger number present themselves for chronic supportive care over a long period of time. The ability to handle these patients in a satisfactory manner remains a very difficult task for most physicians and nurses. The family, who often demonstrates an even more emotional reaction to the patient's illness, can and often does become a trying experience for us. Notwithstanding the psychiatric aspects of many of the problems that these patients bring to the office or clinic, much of their care remains with the treating physician or surgeon and, in recent years, with the nursing profession.

The Patient

Each individual responds in his own characteristic fashion to anything which may threaten or interfere with the normal tenor of his life. Some minimize situations, while some deny the existence of the threat and try to rationalize its cause. Others exaggerate the situation and gain attention by increasing their dependency on others. Still others mobilize anger, blame and defiance of their own ill health while focusing their energy on outside provocation.

On the positive side, health and well-being are expressed in terms of the individual's ability to engage in certain forms of activity that we have come to identify as signifying intactness, safety and a sense of belonging. For example, the heavy laborer may react only slightly to a situation in which difficulty with speech occurs, but in which his muscular system remains intact; a teacher with the same disability may well be precipitated into a severe depressive reaction.

The same striving and defense mechanisms that characterize the intact individual tend to persist in the sick patient. Even facing death, the individual remains more or less true to his basic personality. The person who all his life has shown a tendency to minimize and rationalize in the face of any obstacle, handicap or defect will respond to severe illness by the same denial of the fact that anything is wrong.

It has been suggested since the time of Galen that malignant disease more commonly occurs among persons with a particular psychological make-up. Galen in his treatise *De Tumoribus* observed that melancholic women were more prone to cancer than sanguine women. Others have made similar observations; these have included Ambroise Pare, Alexander Monroe, James Paget and Carl Rokitansky. Recently, Kissen (1) has characterized the personality of the lung cancer patient by stating that a characteristic feature is the poor outlet for emotional discharge.

It is not common for cancer patients to ask outright of the physician, "Do I have cancer?" What is more, patients who do not ask the question usually are not appreciative of the honest physician who volunteers this information. Medically, cancer patients are "good," by which we really mean submissive and cooperative. Rarely do they give doctors and nurses much trouble; the same can be said for children with leukemia. It has been pointed out often that cancer patients are highly dependent persons and are easily addicted to substances like alcohol and tobacco and, of course, to narcotics. Indeed, it has been said that the missing link between tobacco and cancer is the personality which exposes the cells of the mouth, nose, throat and lungs to the carcinogens that exist in tobacco smoke (2).

A typical patient of the author is a French Canadian ex-dock worker who lives with his mother. He has been a heavy smoker for most of his adult life and is a heavy beer drinker. He developed a carcinoma of the larynx and underwent total laryngectomy in a submissive, cooperative manner. He accepted his defect with composure, but still smokes cigarettes through his permanent tracheostomy. He has never worked since his operation although he is a strong, muscular individual. He is very dependent on the clinic and needs to be pampered both by the medical staff and by his aged mother who puts up with the occasional temper tantrums brought on by his excessive drinking.

The tragedy of the incurable patient with far-advanced disease is seen all too frequently. While this may relate solely to the biological activity of the neoplasm itself, more often there has been a delay on the patient's part in seeking medical help. Underlying fear, in spite of all efforts at public education, will unhappily continue to paralyze patients as long as cancer is known to be a catastrophic illness.

When the patient has presented himself for treatment and a diagnosis has been established, the first question which arises is what to tell the patient. This is often paraphrased as "whether or not to tell the truth." Some patients will state outright or imply that they do not want to know what is really wrong, while others suggest that they would like "the truth" in gradual steps rather than all at once. Others, of course, do want to know whether their worst fears are justified, and they may be subjected to even greater anxiety and a sense of distrust if they are told a lie or if they are told different things by different physicians (3). Although doubt remains among the members of the medical profession about whether or not to tell the truth to those persons who ask for it, Kelly and Foriesen (4) found that 89% of 100 cancer patients wanted to be told the truth. However, Oken (1961) surveyed the medical attitudes of the staff of a large hospital in Chicago and found that only 12% of the doctors volunteered to him that they disclose the true facts of the diagnosis if cancer has been found (5).

In the opinion of the author, who has faced this problem for many years, the majority of patients can be told the facts about their illness in a gentle, hopeful manner. No patient should ever be told that his disease is untreatable, and all patients must be given at least some measure of hope. In fact, it is not really relevant to argue whether or not the patient should be told the truth, for one must definitely tell the truth—possibly not all of it at one time—but never anything that is totally untruthful. The patient may be spared the details of an almost certain downward course by employing natural enough methods of circumlocution. The wishes of relatives in this regard can be disturbing for they often feel that the patient will be much happier if told that he has something less serious than a fatal condition. This usually leads to the greatest problem of all—maintaining the original lie, which creates mistrust on the part of everyone.

Feder (6) has stated rightly that many patients complain about the absence of honest and frank communication during the investigative phase of their care. Indeed, the long and uncomfortable "work-up" can be the time of greatest anxiety for patients; they are being examined and probed in every conceivable way and quickly become aware that there is a serious problem. It is still largely unrecognized by both the medical and nursing professions that these early feelings of anxiety and uncertainty must be attended to if more serious sequelae are to be avoided.

Although it is true that one should attempt at this time not to induce psychopathology, one can hardly fail to evoke some intense emotional response from a patient when so much depends on the diagnosis. If too little is told, the original anxiety and fear remain; if too much is told, depression will ensue; it is necessary to steer between these two extremes. One can usually trust the patient to accept the diagnosis with a minimum of emotional response. Indeed, the physician often seems to demonstrate more fear and depression than does the patient. It is well to remember the words of Goethe, "If we take people as they are, we make them worse. If we treat them as if they were what they ought to be, we help them to become that which they are capable of becoming." Notwithstanding this general rule it is wise to be cautious with patients who have had previous mental illness or depression, or who have watched a loved one go through a similar malignant illness.

Normally, the first reaction to the news of a diagnosis of malignant disease is disbelief. The second response is concern regarding treatment. Now one hears, "I'll do anything you say to get well," or "Now that I know what's wrong, what are *we* going to do about it?" Some bolster their morale by saying, "I'm sure it's going to turn out all right because I haven't neglected it."

With this acceptance of the diagnosis, there is a mild reactive depression. The patient must then be given the opportunity to express his fears in his own way, in his own language, and with his own sense of understanding. A good nursing staff is invaluable in this regard, especially if the problems and the need for understanding them have been recognized in advance and plans have been made to deal with them.

Fear underlies virtually all the patient's reactions at this point in his illness. It is perhaps based on the feeling that he or she will be a social outcast. This is often verbalized as "the neighbors" who "will whisper" that so and so "has cancer." At other times, it is the feeling of the patient who is of an independent bent that "everyone is going to feel sorry for me."

Other fears of the patient may be related to pain or suffering or mutilation by surgery. Fears of this sort may be manifested in dreams of a frightening nature before surgery takes place.

The ultimate fear, of course, concerns death. In actuality it is often not death but "abandonment" that is most feared. Death cannot truly be conceptualized, and usually is understood as "aloneness in the face of Eternity." To a large extent religious beliefs color the fears of some patients. There are others who do not want to live, and yet are afraid to die.

The Family

Relatives may react more violently than the patient to the news of a fatal illness. There are a number of common immediate reactions. Initial bewilderment is evidenced by questions such as, "Why did this have to happen to my husband who never hurt anyone in his life and has so much to live for?" The question of course is unanswerable because it is impossible to rationalize this situation.

Shands (7) has pointed out that the news that someone has cancer is greatly complicated in a western world in which rationality has been a general goal for hundreds of years, for cancer seems to be totally irrational and random. Some day it may be possible to make rational sense out of the incidence of malignancy, but for the present "the only sense is the nonsense of statistics." It is still true that "cancer strikes those it strikes, and one cannot say why this one, and not that one." Even in fields where known carcinogens are at work, there is a selection of exposed individuals which cannot be explained. Why, for example, does the majority of even heavy smokers remain well, while a small minority is pushed over the metaphorical precipice by their desire for tobacco? What we human beings find so hard to accept is the casual, the irrational and the unpredictable nature of this process.

Perhaps the impact of tragedy is strongest when a young person is stricken with a fatal disease, for here here is a deeply sensed loss of both present and future happiness. In dealing with parents one finds a mixture of sorrow, pity, love and guilt. Although it is difficult to do so, the allaying of guilt is one of the most important aspects of parent counselling.

The acute anxiety of most relatives lasts one or two weeks, although sometimes it may persist longer. During this period they need definitive help in the form of sympathetic concern, and sometimes sedation to ensure adequate rest. A common reaction is broken sleep with awakenings every hour or two during the night. At each awakening there is automatically the return of thought and sorrow over the patient in the hospital, the diagnosis, and the bleak future.

A second reaction is that of escape. It is frequently seen in an already neurotic personality or in persons with schizoid tendencies. There may be an attempt to find a refuge in alcohol.

A third reaction which can be quite intense is that of acute depression. This may be precipitated by the presence of an underlying guilt. Suddenly, one who has not been fully appreciated may be taken away by death. All the tender emotions come close to the surface; repeated spells of crying are not at all uncommon in both men and women. Although these people certainly require help, they should not be given so-called "mood elevators"; if anything, a mild tranquilizer may help, but even this must not be overdone. Instead, the relative should be allowed to go through the dreadful hours without too much interference, for it generally is better that emotions be expressed fully at this time than be buried only to reappear in later years as a neurotic symptom.

Another reaction of persons who feel guilt is the repeated, and at times foolish, buying of gifts for the patient in the hospital. By this behavior they are trying to say that they will now "make up for all those years when I did so little."

The Post-Operative Patient

There are certain immediate post-operative psychological states that are readily recognized. Adsett (8) has summarized a number which are found in the patient who has just had a cancer operation. As these are of great importance to the attending medical and nursing staff, they seem worthy of discussion at this point.

1. Most patients exhibit *regression*. This is a natural return to the dependency of childhood. The patient is anxious, helpless, childlike, and may complain about a lack of attention or sympathy. While this attitude should be tolerated for a day or two, the staff must try to make a point of not allowing it to become chronic. As soon as possible, the patient should be made to do as much for himself as possible.

2. *Anxiety* is found either alone or in association with other symptoms. It should be understood that as a result of surgery there has been a sudden change in body image. There is often the fear of unacceptability or perhaps even rejection by husband, wife or close friends. This is most commonly seen after operations on the breast, uterus, vagina, penis, or face, or in patients who have previously used physical and sexual attractiveness as the basis for admiration, friendship or marriage.

3. *Depression* follows a sense of loss. This includes the feeling of body loss in a somatic sense, as well as loss of the life activities associated with loss of a specific organ. Again this is most commonly seen after operations on sexual organs; it also occurs in persons whose sense of worth through performing services for others has been interrupted.

The symptoms of depression are protean in nature, but usually are associated with feelings of worthlessness. The patient is unable to read or concentrate on anything for more than a few minutes. If there is underlying guilt, he/she may be tearful. In some instances one may hear, "I wish I had died on the operating table," or "I wish I did not have to wake up tomorrow morning." However, it is rare to hear anything which suggests actual suicide.

4. *Hostility* is quite common. Although the surgeon may be seen as the injuring person, out of fear of "retaliation" resentment may be displaced to members of the family or the nursing staff. Sometimes when patients seem to be demonstrating paranoid tendencies, they are in fact only projecting their anger. They may, for example, suspect that there was a mistake in the diagnosis, or that treatment was much too extensive or even unnecessary.

It is important to realize that there is usually nothing personal about this hostility, and that expressed anger is better than self-directed hostility. In the long run, the hostile patient often does very well.

5. *Hypochondriasis* can be an association of depression and paranoia. It appears in masochistic individuals who have an underlying self-destructive tendency and hostility towards those responsible for their present state. They fully expect to be left with residual, permanent injury. They see their bodies as forever weakened, and their lives as never again approaching normality. The reaction is quite common in women after operations on the ovaries or uterus, and in many men after orchidectomy. The prognosis is usually poor.

6. *Counterphobia* is, in simple terms, "bravado" behavior. It leads to inappropriate and foolish attempts to prove that neither the illness nor the operation is "going to get me down." Such patients should be told that they must allow their bodies a period of convalescence and rest. It is important to realize that "bravado" behavior is almost always a veneer over fear and depression.

7. *Obsessive compulsive reactions* usually result after operations on the urinary or rectal sphincters, especially when ileal conduits have been fashioned or colostomies instituted. In our modern society, acts of excretion are prohibited as subjects for conversation and certainly not demonstrable in front of others. There is nothing so private in our day and age as the bathroom! With artificial bladders or colostomies, patients live in constant fear of "spillage," and are mortified by the sound of escaping gas and the odor that may result.

8. *Schizophrenia or post-operative panic.* Mastrovito (9) recently has dealt with this subject in an extensive manner. This type of acute reaction generally occurs within the first week of the post-operative period, although it can manifest itself as late as two or three weeks after operation, or as early as a few hours after awakening in the recovery room.

These panics are sudden and dramatic for all concerned. The patient can turn abruptly into a hostile, suspicious, delusional and hallucinating individual. The delusions are paranoid, with the patient attributing malevolence to the actions of the hospital staff. When present, hallucinations are almost always auditory and the content is threatening, frightening and damning.

Prodromal signs are few. Several days prior to the onset of the illness, the patient may spend restless nights and during the day may seem surly, hostile or less communicative than usual. The onset of the panic state is invariably accompanied by a marked and sudden rise in pulse rate, and in about one-third of the cases this phenomenon occurs almost twenty-four hours in advance of the actual acute episode. The need for medication is immediate. Barbiturates, mild tranquilizers and hypnotics, while not necessarily contraindicated, are usually not desirable. The treatment of choice rests with the class of drugs under the general title of the phenothiazines. Chlorpromazine, thorazine (R), or largactil (R) are effective if given in large doses by intramuscular injection every two to six hours. Regardless of apparent improvement, a pulse rate that has not dropped during this period is an indication that too little drug has been given.

The physician should not overlook the need to allay anxiety experienced by the nursing staff and other ward personnel. Special nurses must be assigned around the clock. Visits from friends, family, members of the clergy, and others should be severely restricted. Nursing and medical procedures must be performed in a manner that insures minimal misinterpretation by the patient. For example, the nurse should accompany all her ministrations with explanations about what she is going to do, and for what purpose. All procedures should be carried out directly in front of the patient or entirely out of his presence. Conversations at the bedside should be conducted in a loud enough manner for the patient to hear clearly. Whispering must be avoided at all cost.

Children

In dealing with children, honesty on the part of the medical and nursing staff is imperative. It is likewise important to persuade the parents that they too should remain honest about what the child is told. Breaks in communication, or statements that vary from one adult to another, lead only to lack of trust and security on the part of the child who then continues to live in constant doubt and fear.

When a child is old enough to know the meaning of words, he should be told what is being planned. This is especially true in the traumatic situation where a limb or even an eye has to be removed. To have a child forewarned is infinitely better than trying to deal with the young patient who awakens from his anesthetic to realize that he can no longer walk or see.

Children always want to know what "will hurt." If a particular ministration is going to be painful, the child should be so informed. When something is relatively painless, he can also be told so in advance. In this way, the child's trust is built up and reinforced. Children, with their very active imaginations and fears, invariably accept more readily fact than frightening fantasy.

The Incurable Patient

When illness is recurrent or there has been metastatic spread from a previously excised carcinoma, there are new sets of reactions both in the patient and in the family. The initial hopes for total cure have now faded, and there is general sorrow on the part of the patient. In addition, there are anxieties of various kinds about the family situation in the absence of the patient. Occasionally one finds resentment against religious belief; this is understandable when it is realized that during the previous months or years the patient, his family and friends have been praying for his health and recovery. Suddenly it appears that prayer has been of no avail, and a feeling of skepticism takes over.

By this time the spirit of independence usually has left the patient and he becomes quite dependent on his physician. Now more than at any other time the patient needs an advisor he can trust; one who will ameliorate the illness, be near and available when help is needed, make sure that he does not suffer too much, and will allow him to die with dignity.

The hospital staff often has trouble understanding the needs of such patients, for they see the disease as hopeless and the patient as one condemned to die in the near future. Friends, too, often find it difficult to talk to such persons. If there has been acceptance of the patient on a hospital ward, the patient may demonstrate the unfortunate side effect of dependency on the staff for both physical and psychological comfort. Such patients should be seen by a competent team of doctors and nurses in an out-patient department where they can be given frequent appointments, and the "right" to telephone from home if something is worrying them.

This "telephone talk" and office visits for psychological needs rather than physical needs can keep a specially trained secretary and good graduate nurse busy for a large part of the day. On a large unit, perhaps three or four trained paramedical members are required to meet these needs. It is usually a good idea for each patient to be introduced as early as possible to all members of the "team," so he will have the assurance that someone he knows will be available whenever he calls. This is particularly important for those patients who are "public" or "charity," for they rarely have a personal physician who can be called on a Saturday afternoon, and are otherwise faced with the prospect of turning up at an emergency department where they will be seen by an intern or resident who has no knowledge of the case.

Many patients are often self-centered and suspicious at the beginning of treatment, but a cheerful and sympathetic approach on the part of the whole team will usually rectify this. Some patients, however, remain self-centered and selfish, especially when in their own homes, and many remain depressed. Only rarely are qualified psychiatrists called in. Rather the hospital team, with the assistance of a good social worker, and often the invaluable help of a member of the nursing profession who can see the patient at home, tries to stimulate or maintain the interest of the patient in one or several of a long list of activities. These might include returning to work; travel, if the patient is able and has sufficient financial resources; reading; gardening; care of a pet or birds that are lured to the patient's window by some seed. For others, films or television can prove most useful.

Even when it is obvious to the members of the medical staff that they are dealing with an incurable condition which can at best be palliated for a few months, some degree of hope must be maintained. It has been said that "hope should not die too far ahead of the patient." It may be hope of getting better, but often it is only the hope of the enjoyment of conversation with relatives or grandchildren tomorrow, or even the hope that appetite may improve in a few days. Mood elevators may now help to moderate the underlying impatience at the length of the illness and the patient's continuing weakness.

It is unkind to tell a patient who has to be hospitalized for complications of his recurrent or metastatic carcinoma that he will soon be all right. It is better to state the specific goal soon after admission and that the aim is to have the patient home in a certain number of days. The patient should be warned that, on the other hand, various tests or X-rays may disclose problems that are not immediately suspected, and that these too may have to be looked after or treated.

When death obviously is near, most patients become apathetic and disinterested in abstract values. Nor is there much to be gained by trying to discuss the weather, the news or even stories about the family. Too much emphasis on food intake, fluids, bathing or hair care is irritating rather than comforting. It would seem that in all beings there is the curious knowledge of impending dissolution or death. This strange foresight is manifested consciously as withdrawal and lack of concentration on things of the moment.

Nurses and doctors at this stage often find great difficulty in communicating with the patient. Indeed, as Rothenberg (10) has pointed out, many physicians resist identification with dying patients and may even wish that the patient would "hurry up and die." These wishes are then rationalized on the grounds that the patient is "suffering such pain." Often the patient recognizes this attitude, and the physician then withdraws further, and discourages discussion or any sort of emotional interaction. Rothenberg (10) also studied the factors operating between typical hospital house staff and terminal cancer patients. He found that staff members tended to support patient denial, encouraged isolation, discouraged the expression of grief, overestimated the patient's incapacity because of their own sense of failure, and avoided issues that made manifest the fact of loss of control. On the other hand, the staff may sometimes persist in being cheerful and by this attitude deny the knowledge of impending death. In other words, they persist in minimizing to the patient the gravity of a situation that is fully realized by the patient himself. This unfortunately destroys the patient's faith in the staff and at the same time makes it difficult for him to deal with the situation realistically or honestly.

A dying person fears desertion above all else. He is now incapable of standing and fighting alone, and this is realized either consciously or unconsciously. His life has been full of experiences both happy and unhappy, but no matter how long or short that life has been, it has been coped with as he thought best. To protect themselves from being ignored, patients may use attention-seeking mechanisms such as sleeplessness or idle "chattiness." If medical and nursing personnel do not meet these needs, "demanding behavior" will become all the more common.

Possibly the most helpful way in which the staff can communicate with a patient is simply to meet him on his own ground. The dying patient concentrates on the pain, the appetite, the weakness or dizziness of the moment. This, then, is the plane of communication. "I see that you finished your breakfast this morning—that's an improvement over yesterday!" or, "What a shame that you could not finish your lunch today—but you know how days change. Tomorrow, lunch (or dinner) will probably be better." "Remember that your body is good at knowing what it needs— if you feel sleepy, then rest; when you wake up, you might feel like a snack." Thus each tiny aspect of the day is a goal. If met and overcome, it becomes a great success; if missed, it is compared with yesterday, or the hope of tomorrow. Unfavorable comparisons may precipitate a depression that is difficult to handle. To avert this it should be borne in mind at all times that goals must be realistic.

Some physicians and nurses feel that this approach is a sham, in that they know that any small victory will in no way affect the inevitable outcome. Let us be aware that the patient is not being fooled; he realizes that the end is near. Nevertheless, he needs objectives and rewards. When the future is limited, objectives are proportionately limited, but they nevertheless are as important as they ever were.

An important although small point should perhaps be interjected here. Caring for dying patients creates a certain strain on personnel, and it is most important to understand staff needs as well as patient needs. The physician or the nurse who must treat cancer patients day in and day out needs to be strengthened and reassured by easy, free, less defensive communication with his or her peers and seniors.

As death nears, control of pain and allaying of anxiety are the primary goals. Some patients fear taking too much analgesic. It is thus important to observe carefully for the unspoken signs of pain—restlessness, sweating and irritability. These patients must be asked if they have pain. If it is explained that tolerance of pain will not improve the condition, pain-relieving compounds may be more readily acceptable (11). Furthermore, it is true that a patient in pain does not expand his lungs as well as possible, does not eat as well as he could, or does not move about in the bed or get up into a chair as he might otherwise be able. Controlling pain is always a worthwhile step.

There is always sympathy for a patient at this juncture and there should be empathy. Unfortunately the training in modern medical institutions seems to teach only the exploitation of grief for the purpose of obtaining a post-mortem examination! While doctors should know more about dying and death than any other men, too many of us seem to think no more of it than the full stop at the end of a moving novel. Like Sartre we seem to believe that "death is not inherent in life." It could be said that we have become desensitized to the symbols of death and are trying to convince others that we have no inner fear.

There is most certainly room for self-criticism within our profession, for it seems that we physicians are less suited than are others to face the care of the dying; indeed these terminal patients are a symbol of our incompetence as we pursue an idealized art of healing (12). Instead of feeding our narcissism by responding and getting well, these dying patients and their relatives are demanding and frustrating. This is not to say that we are consciously neglectful, but it is a true that in our larger hospitals pre-terminal patients and their families are rarely approached with any sense of sympathy or even interest (13). Meanwhile, we keep ourselves busy and deny the reality of death. It is all too true that we hide—behind a couch, a surgeon's mask, or a pose of "intellectualization."

Although our disillusionment with our competency may show up as sympathy, it may show itself equally to the patient and the family as anger, disappointment, embarrassment or worse, indifference. Sorrow, pity and sympathy which are only counter-transference from our patients, are supportive to the dying not only because the patient feels love, but perhaps because he senses that we, the whole members of society, can be made more human by our kindnesses toward the failing. We are all helped when we recognize our own fears, weaknesses and the reality of our hopes. Knowledge of our own human condition may soften the blows of our failures and disillusionments.

Most modern families with a dying relative realize that everything which medical science has to offer has been tried. A few families may want another consultant, and some may want to show the doctors and nurses a magazine or a newspaper clipping that extols a new "miracle" treatment. These should always be taken and read with sympathy, and a sensible explanation given as to why the treatment would not help. Occasionally there are anguished pleas not to let the patient die, but the grieving family should be helped to accept the fact of coming loss.

If an "explanation" of the death is demanded, it is wise to understand the religious orientation of the family before answering. The author has developed different types of "explanations" for those who do, or do not, believe in an afterlife, and have varying concepts of a Creator. This point need not be elaborated, and is mentioned only to re-emphasize the meaning of the word "sympathy." One cannot "feel with" the patient if one is ignorant of the basic concept on which the patient's life has been lived. Medically speaking, it is usually enough to say to the family that the patient, were he to live, or had he lived, would have been a cripple in terms of lungs, heart, liver, kidney or brain, or would never have been relieved completely of pain or suffering.

Death can often be seen as a friend rather than as the classic "grim reaper" with which the medical and nursing professions are supposedly in constant conflict. Just as we help people into this world, we must also help them as they leave it.

References

1. D. M. Kissen, "The Significance of Personality in Lung Cancer in Men," *Annals of the New York Academy of Sciences, 125,* 1966.

2. J. G. Henderson, E. Witthower, and M. N. Lougheed, "A Psychiatric Investigation of the Delay Factor in Patients to Doctor Presentation in Cancer," *Journal of Psychosomatic Research, 3,* 1958.

3. C. S. Cameron, *Medical News,* August 31, 1960.

4. W. D. Kelly and S. R. Foriesen, "Do Cancer Patients Want to Be Told?", *Surgery, 27,* 1950.

5. D. Oken, "What to Tell Cancer Patients: A Study of Medical Attitudes," *Journal of the American Medical Association, 75,* 1961.

6. S. L. Feder, "Psychological Considerations in the Case of Patients with Cancer," *Annals of the New York Academy of Sciences, 125,* 1966.

7. H. C. Shands, "The Information Aspect of Cancer on the Structure of the Human Personality," *Annals of the New York Academy of Sciences, 125,* 1966.

8. C. S. Adsett, "Emotional Reactions to Disfigurement from Cancer Chemotherapy," *Canadian Medical Association Journal, 89,* August 1963.

9. R. C. Mastrovito, "Acute Psychological Problems and the Use of Psychotropic Medicines in the Treatment of Cancer Patients," *Annals of the New York Academy of Sciences, 125,* 1966.

10. A Rothenberg, "Psychological Problems in Terminal Cancer Management," *Cancer, 14,* 1961.

11. H. H. Garner, *Psychosomatic Management of the Patient with Malignancy.* Springfield, Illinois: Charles C. Thomas, 1966.

12. B. Schoenberg, A. C. Carr, D. Peretz, and A. H. Kutscher (Eds.), *Loss and Grief: Psychological Management in Medical Practice.* New York: Columbia University Press, 1970.

13. E. Kubler-Ross, *On Death and Dying.* New York: The Macmillan Company, 1970.

The Oral System in *Bereavement*

*David Peretz**

Reaction to the real or threatened loss of a loved person, possession or function is often profound and in some cases takes on the nature of an illness. It represents a significant departure from the person's usual state of feeling, thinking and behavior, and may be accompanied by physical and emotional symptoms. Such reactions are referred to as bereavement reactions or states and range from the "normal" grief reaction which is limited in intensity and duration to more extended, debilitating and chronic states. The latter are exaggerated, persistent, and can be crippling and disruptive to the bereaved, his family and friends. Certain bereavement states may give the appearance of being adaptive with no apparent symptoms of grief, yet the absence of a reaction in the context of a significant loss itself may be a harbinger of future maladaptation.

Varieties of bereavement states include:

> grief
> anticipatory grief
> inhibited, delayed and absent grief
> chronic grief
> depression
> hypochondriasis and exacerbation of pre-existent somatic conditions
> development of medical symptoms and illness
> psychophysiologic reactions.
> drug usage, promiscuity or appearance of psychopathic behavior
> specific neurotic and psychotic states (i.e., conversion reaction, psychotic depression, etc.) (1)

Recently, both clinical data and research evidence have suggested that "the death of or separation from a loved one is a critical factor in the development of a broad variety of somatic disturbances, including fatal illness. Disorders mentioned in the literature include cancer, tuberculosis,

---

*Department of Psychiatry, College of Physicians and Surgeons, Columbia University, New York, New York.

ulcerative colitis, asthma, obesity, thyrotoxicosis and diabetes mellitus." Schoenberg and Carr have demonstrated the relation between loss and specific oral complaints, i.e., the burning mouth syndrome (2).

The mouth may become involved to a greater or lesser extent in bereavement states through mechanisms to be described in the following discussion.

Early in life, the mouth is involved in activities which, by mediating survival needs, reduction of tension, production and repetition of pleasure, attachment to loved objects through communication, and discharge of aggression, come to be variously represented in our mental world, often with high emotional valence. By its early, repetitive and crucial role in the above activities, the mouth also readily becomes a normal site for fantasy of a wide variety. Each person integrates the mouth apparatus in a characteristic way. Constitutional or temperament factors (such as the level of oral drives, i.e., sucking, biting, chewing, mouthing), traumatic experiences (early illness involving face or mouth, unusual deprivations or frustrations, excessive stimulation) as well as normal experiential factors interact in unique ways for each of us, determining the nature and outcome of this "mouth integration." Imitation of and identification with significant persons in early as well as later life may lead the individual to attach particular significance to the mouth and face. Social and cultural factors, as well, play a facilitating role as releasors or inhibitors of particular mouth modes, mediated first through primary objects and later through various figures in the environment.

The mouth appears to become both site and mode for an early understanding of the mysteries of the world by the growing small child. In mental representations of the small child, pregnancy, for example, is often associated with oral incorporation. We can see the strength of oral needs manifested in adult sexual and non-sexual behaviors in many individuals, with much inter-individual variation. We can also see defenses against these needs or impulses exhibited by individuals and societies in the condemnation and shame attached to oral practices, particularly sexual ones. That mouth, tongue and lips function as erogenous areas can be seen in the role of sucking, biting, licking and kissing in sexual activity, while non-sexual representations of mouth activity range from eating to speaking to smoking to expressing emotionality.

Some of the earliest losses occur in and around the mouth: weaning from breast or bottle, loss of baby teeth, giving up voluntarily or under coercion the thumb or other "mouthing" objects, the ultimate failure (earlier or later, depending upon circumstances) of crying (via the mouth) to bring the tension relieving object immediately or quickly to provide satisfaction. Again, there is a complementary relation between the time of the experience, the nature and capacity of the individual in its drives, defenses and ego-strength, the quality and availability of the caring object, and the trauma that will determine the character and adaptiveness of mouth integration. The nature and content of these early experiences will also provide the matrix if regression should occur in later life in response to frustration or loss.

With these facts in mind, it is not difficult to understand the finding that "of patients exposed to various degrees of trauma, a larger number experience conscious fear with minor dental procedures than when confronted with major surgery on other parts of the body (3)." Extraction of teeth may be viewed unconsciously as castrations, bodily mutilation or death. Bleeding from the oral cavity may be connected with abortion, sexual invasion or rape (4).

Emotional needs may be expressed in some individuals to a significant degree through the face and mouth. Facial expressions, mouth expressions, rate, flow and volume of speech, emotionality of speech, use of tongue are but a few of these pathways of discharge. The teeth are clearly involved in these processes as well. Characteristically or only at times, individuals may defend themselves against expressing emotionality through the face and mouth (increased muscle tone, rigidity of expression, clenching teeth, pursing lips, and so on).

The anticipated or actual loss of something highly valued acts as a danger signal. The outcome of this loss depends upon our capacity to anticipate realistically the loss and its meaning and to mobilize effective coping mechanisms. When loss is anticipated or has already occurred, many people may demonstrate *regressive* maneuvers. These may be benign or more serious in their implications for health. Mental functioning, in regression, moves back to earlier representations of object-relations, defenses, and more "primitive," less sublimated drive-representations; that is, to earlier ways of thinking, feeling, acting, perceiving and expressing. Within the dental situation, the behavior of a person who has visited the dentist's office previously and now comes in for a repetition of a simple procedure filled with tension will probably exhibit regression at some level. The regressive unconscious imagery may be managed by a number of defenses—the patient may use rationalization and intellectualization or may deny the symptoms, or repress the appointment, or see the dentist as cruel rather than seeing himself as frightened of a situation in which he is helpless.

Death has a particular capacity to promote regressive structures. If it is the death of a loved one or part of oneself, need-fulfilling gratification is threatened in fantasy or actuality. To the extent that regression occurs in response to the loss, mouth integration may also regress (not only in terms of actual behavior with the mouth, but also fantasied activity with mouth - sucking, licking, biting and the associated old emotionality and defense). One's fear of his own death may also be mobilized.

Bereavement is a state, then, in which "tension" is likely to be high. The associated regressions, as well as the repairs that accompany them in an attempt to adapt to the loss or anticipated loss, are associated with non-specific and specific mechanisms that can relate to the oral system.

In dealing with the bereaved, we may be confronted with individuals who have a normal oral system, those whose oral system is marginal (the predisposed), or those with a definite history of oral pathology.

Non-specific mechanisms which may occur in bereavement include the following:
>   neglect of oral care
>   misuse of the oral system (biting, clenching, grinding, changed dietary practices, increase in smoking, use of drugs with adverse effect on the oral system)
>   demand for painful procedures to discharge unconscious guilt associated with bereavement reaction

Specific reactions which may occur in bereavement include the following:
1. conversion (i.e., hysterical or atypical facial pain): a painful affect is given symbolic expression through a compliant somatic symptom
2. affective equivalents: instead of direct, subjective experience of anxiety or depression, somatic symptoms associated with the affect occur (i.e., bruxism, muscular tension, burning tongue)
3. depression: may lead to non-specific mechanisms, above equivalents or even to delusional ideas about the mouth (poisoning, foul smell, etc.—in psychotic depression. Change in salivary function may be reflected in associated dry mouth, etc.)

4. hypochondriasis: the elaboration of a minor oral problem or minor effects of dental procedures to the status of a major preoccupation—the patient may be convinced that a dread disease is present
5. other neurotic and psychotic mechanisms

Oral pathology may also occur in bereavement states (e.g., dry mouth may result from antidepressant or tranquilizer medication).

Identification with the lost loved object may occur in the bereavement state: if the lost person had pronounced oral symptoms before or during the terminal illness, there may be manifestation of similar symptoms in the bereaved. Similarly, if an earlier important person who was lost had oral symptoms or disease, the loss may renew early identification and the bereaved may take on those symptoms.

Concluding Remarks

The medical or dental personnel who would provide oral care for the bereaved initially must increase their sensitivity to the role of loss or threatened loss in the pathogenesis of oral disorders. Physicians probably pay less attention to the oral system, unless it presents acutely, than to many other systems. Medical history is not often keyed to inquire into oral pathology involving lips, gums, teeth, tongue, buccal mucosa and the state of the anterior portions of the oral cavity. Subtle symptoms of early oral pathology may be overlooked. When the bereaved does present to the physician or dentist with oral complaints, it is the responsibility of the doctor to make careful inquiry about recent losses and to listen with care to the patient for associated emotional states. It may then become apparent that the primary problem is in the nature of the bereavement reaction and the patient and doctor may be spared the problems arising out of dental procedures performed electively in the bereaved. There is reason to suggest that during periods of bereavement, elective dental extraction and other operative procedures should be delayed to permit the bereavement process to run its course, if medical and dental indications permit.

The dental history should include the identification of recent or threatened loss, the cause of the loss, and whether oral system pathology was present at some point in the history of the loved person. Were there other earlier losses of valued or loved objects and what part did the mouth play in those losses? A careful family history will elicit this data and can be accomplished in a routine way. To be able to take such a history requires that the interviewer be prepared to accept the emotional expression that the bereaved may put forth. Often, in order to avoid the painful feelings engendered in us in sharing the feelings of the bereaved, we subtly organize our approach to the patient to prevent such expression. Such an approach only causes the patient to seek out another dentist/physician ostensibly for additional oral treatment, but actually for someone who will listen and offer emotional support.

The history should also include an inquiry into the mechanics of utilization of the oral system and related emotional function. For example, how and when does one chew, bite (pencils, fingers, food), is it done slowly or rapidly, sucking (thumb, bone, food), or suppression of these responses.

The mouth, as an organ system, is amenable do direct observation. Its vascular state, dryness or moistness, color, and so on, can be viewed by the examiner. It is true that observation of the mouth requires that it be open, which immediately reduces its capacity to function in communication. The dentist must communicate with the patient at a time separate from the treatment itself. This may reduce the possibility of observing fully the relationship between the oral system and its function and importance to that patient. Effective communication in the dental situation often centers around anticipation of the procedures or consequences of the producers.

Many important questions about the mouth in bereavement remain unanswered while others have not yet been asked. It is hoped that increased attention and study of the oral system under this major, ubiquitous stress will contribute to our knowledge of the psychophysiology and dynamic aspects of the oral cavity.

References

1. D. Peretz, "Reaction to Loss," chapter in *Loss and Grief: Psychological Management in Medical Practice*, edited by B. Schoenberg, A. C. Carr, D. Peretz, and A. H. Kutscher, New York: Columbia University Press, 1970.

2. A. C. Carr and B. Schoenberg, "Object-Loss and Somatic Symptom Formation," *Loss and Grief: Psychological Management in Medical Practice*.

3. *Ibid*.

4. A. H. Kutscher and B. Schoenberg, "Special Considerations Regarding Tooth Extractions in Grief and Depression," *Dental Clinics of North America*, October 1969, p. 967.

SELECTED MEDICAL SPECIALTIES

Internal Medicine and the Oral Care of the Dying Patient

Manuel Ochoa, Jr.*

The dying patient may suffer from the oral manifestations of a systemic disease or the terminal aspects of a disease of the mouth and adnexa. The maintenance of the highest level of oral hygiene, an essential objective in the care of the dying patient, is attained by integrated attention to the total needs of the patient. Terminal disease, be it systemic or local, may produce profound alterations in the oral environment: xerostomia, periodontitis and carious lesions; the categories include all known pathophysiological entities. These alterations may adversely influence general physical functions and the deterioration of the latter, in turn, further exacerbates the deterioration of the condition of the oral cavity. Moreover, oral care of the dying patient should not be restricted to the treatment of physical disabilities. Maintenance of the highest level of oral hygiene may subserve the emotional needs of the individual and facilitate social intercourse.

Dietary and Nutritional Problems

Feeding the dying patient is frequently a major problem. Malnutrition and weight loss are important complications of treatment. The malnourished and debilitated patient is affected by cachexia, a syndrome characterized by weakness, anorexia, depletion of host components, electrolyte and water abnormalities, and a progressive fading of vital functions. Besides these symptoms, more subtle manifestations such as apathy, detachment, and anxiety are well known characteristics. These latter characteristics represent the participation of the mind in the gradual disruption of metabolic processes and in oncoming death.

It appears that protein loss is a major factor in cachexia. It is unknown whether the protein loss is a depletion of body nitrogen or a reflection of an inability to assimilate and use nitrogen in protein synthesis due to metabolic interference. Fat loss is generalized. There are disproportionate losses of minerals relative to that of sodium; elevated serum copper concentrations have also been described, as have water abnormalities.

---

* Memorial Hospital for Cancer and Allied Diseases, New York, New York

In addition, the dying patient may have a physical impediment to the passage of food (e.g., tumor, fistula, palsy). Frequently, he has infection and fever. Blood loss and the effects of surgery, radiation, and drugs further contribute to anorexia and impair his nutritional status. Under these circumstances, it is understandable that good nutrition, vitamin supplementation, or high protein diets are universally employed as adjuncts to treatment. The chronology and direction of dietary therapy will depend upon the condition of the patient. The dying patient need not be, *a priori,* denied surgery or other procedures. Preoperative improvement in nutrition, where feasible, is essential to insure that the patient is in the best condition to tolerate and recover from such measures as surgery, radiotherapy, or chemotherapy. For example, hypoproteinemia causes a sensitivity to saline solutions, prolongs intestinal transit time, delays wound healing, depresses marrow activity, and reduces antibody formation. It is, therefore, clear that the maintenance of the patient's nutritional state is important.

A series of possibilities should be evaluated. If there is a loss of essential tissue stores, as evidence of a chronically insufficient caloric intake, body fat and protein will be metabolized; therefore, replacement of protein materials (e.g., with Protenium) either orally or parenterally should be "covered" by simultaneous administration of adequate carbohydrates in order to prevent protein utilization for energy metabolism. The questions of adequate amounts of calories and adequate protein supply are important. The protein must possess all essential amino acids in proper balance.

If the patient has anemia, it must be corrected before protein reserves can be fully restored since erythrocyte formation takes precedence over protein disposition. Water intake must be adequate since chronic dehydration, especially in the face of high protein intake, can lead to azotemia. Proper and sufficient intake of calcium, potassium, and magnesium are necessary in order to maintain a favorable milieu for anabolism. Potassium and phosphate are deposited with glycogen, and protein synthesis does not proceed when there is a deficiency of potassium. The specific kinds and amounts of vitamins supplied to the patient during long periods of intravenous, forced oral, or tube feeding must be adequate. Members of the vitamin B complex act as enzymes for various intermediate pathways of metabolism, and the needs for thiamine relate to carbohydrate metabolism. Additional ascorbic acid may be required where demands for wound healing are high and where hypermetabolism, as in continued fever, accelerates depletion of ascorbic acid.

Paradoxically, intense efforts to increase the caloric intake of the patient may have adverse effects. Substantial supplements between meals may only serve to discourage eating at mealtime. However, an additional feeding at bedtime is often advisable. If only small amounts can be eaten at one time, more frequent small meals may be helpful. Meals should be prepared tastefully and served in as enticing a manner as possible. An alcoholic drink taken 15 to 30 minutes before meals may also serve as a stimulant. If eating is painful, a mild narcotic given 30 minutes before meals may permit greater comfort. Adequate sleep and rest are essential.

Parental feeding may be instituted to maintain fluid and electrolyte balance temporarily, and to prevent starvation and negative nitrogen balance. In addition to five per cent glucose, fluid and calories can be given by an intravenous infusion of alcohol (six per cent) or fat emulsions. The latter should not be given regularly for more than two weeks. Protein hydrolysates (Amigen) may be given in five per cent glucose solution. Parenteral feeding, supplying 1,600 calories, supplies considerably less than the normal requirement of 2,500 to 3,000 calories for a hospitalized patient. It has been estimated that at least 2,800 calories a day should be provided so that protein, rather than caloric energy, can be used for anabolism. The difficulty of providing sufficient calories through parenteral feeding alone is obvious.

Diets

Liquid Diet. The patient unable to eat should be fed by tube. The choice of the tube will depend on the condition of the patient and his particular eating problem. Pain on swallowing may be averted by employing a nasal feeding tube, a procedure which many patients can learn to use. For the patient who cannot manage a soft diet, a liquid diet can be used temporarily. A clear liquid diet is highly inadequate, should be considered primarily as fluid replacement, and should be used only until the patient can be placed on an adequate soft diet. A high calorie, high protein, high calcium liquid formula can be used either for supplementation or tube feeding. This is a concentrated milk formulation consisting of 350 gm of dried skim milk added to 730 gm of whole milk, flavored to taste, and diluted as desired.

Soft Diet. A completely soft diet, in liquid form, which is close to nutritional adequacy can be prepared from the following:
one cup of cereal
two eggs
two tablespoons of butter

½ cup of ice cream
one quart of milk
one cup of strained meats
one cup of strained vegetables
½ cup of strained fruit
one quart of fruit juice
one cup of soup

The most appetizing way to serve these strained or pureed foods for three daily servings is to place fruits in fruit juice, meats in soup, and cereal or vegetables in milk, and mix throughly. Variations can be used to suit the patient's taste. Total caloric intake can be increased by increasing quantities or by *ad lib* feedings of milk shakes, egg nogs, and commercially prepared supplemental foods such as Sustagen or Meritene.

The usual hospital soft diet uses low fiber vegetables, tender meats, fruits, and fruit juices. Chopped meats can be triple ground, soups strained, and vegetables pureed, if necessary. Such a low roughage diet is, however, usually inadequate for prolonged use.

Variety can be accomplished through the use of readily available baby foods. These may be most helpful for the outpatient. Each small pureed or strained jar contains 100 gm; meats supply between 100 and 200 calories. Protein and fat can be increased by the addition of whole milk. Protein can also be augmented through the addition of skim milk or meat; and fat through the use of limited amounts of butter, margarine, or liquid fat. Although fat gives the largest caloric increase per gram, the amount to be given the patient is limited by reduction in palatability, particularly if it is added to a cold dish.

A major disadvantage of the use of any single formulation is the length of time that many patients are restricted to special diets. In addition, ease of preparation is particularly important to those patients spending considerable time outside the hospital.

Probably, the best means of attaining a satisfactory diet is to display the whole food on a tray and allow the patient to select what he wishes. The food is then placed in a blender and liquefied, to be eaten or fed by tube. Some patients prefer to first chew the whole food before spitting it into the blender. Serving whole food, as selected by the patient's ethnic, religious, and cultural background, is psychologically very effective since the further preparation changes only its consistency. Any outpatient can be given supervised free choice of food, provided he is willing to use a blender, to mash, grind, strain, and soften food with milk, soup, fruit juice, or gravy.

Supplementation. Vitamin supplementation should be given in therapeutic doses. It is often assumed that all dying patients are somewhat nutritionally depleted but adequate clinical data are not available.

If the patient is anemic, iron should be given either parenterally or perorally. Ascorbic acid helps maintain the iron in reduced form and may promote absorption. Ferrous sulfate (0.3 gm) and ascorbic acid (50 mg) are satisfactory. Additional vitamin C, up to 1 gm daily, is frequently given in the first few days after surgery. This is based on the demonstrated role (in animal studies) of vitamin C in collagen synthesis and its effect in increasing the tensile strength of wounds. Recent studies of collagen biosynthesis in human wound healing have shown that the collagen concentration of connective tissue rises sharply between the second and third week, and then slowly returns to normal. However, it has been shown that it is not back to presurgical levels even at the end of eight weeks.

The patient handicapped by anatomical loss may develop a psychological problem, feeling that eating is virtually impossible. This patient needs reassurance so that he may discover that adequate eating is possible. Occasionally, a patient with severe malaise may show dramatic improvement after adequate feeding.

The soft diet in liquid form described previously consists of about 1½ quarts of liquid per meal. This is often about the capacity of the stomach, although it is sometimes less. As a result the liquid may become isotonic and be rapidly discharged from the stomach, causing the patient to complain of hunger shortly afterwards. More frequent, smaller servings may be helpful in overcoming this problem. An increase in the fat content of the food may also help the stomach to retain its contents for a longer period through the enterogastrone mechanism. In some cases, the addition of methylcellulose to increase bulk is helpful.

An abrupt change in diet frequently causes either constipation or diarrhea. When diarrhea occurs, the composition of the feeding mixture should be checked for an excess of carbohydrate or fat. If the mixture is not at fault, the size and frequency of the feedings should be decreased. Tincture of opium also affords relief. Prune juice, because of its high potassium content, can cause intestinal motility and diarrhea. Therefore, it should be used judiciously. In patients who suffer peristaltic spasms, anticholinergic drugs (Pro-Banthine 30 mg orally) may be employed; Dulcolax may be useful for constipation.

In palliation, anabolic agents may be of value. The anabolic effect of androgens is probably related to nitrogen but also causes retention of potassium, phosphorus, and calcium. On the other hand, however, the androgens cause androgenicity, sodium and water retention, and hepatitis. Norethandrolone (Nilevar) is an agent in which the androgenic effects have been separated from the metabolic effects. The usual dosage is 25 mg t.i.d. Androgen therapy usually demonstrates limited beneficial effects and is not a substitute for food or a well-balanced, vitamin supplemented diet.

Increased frequency of liquid intake is highly desirable, particularly for those patients with a "dry mouth" and its associated problems. Dry, bulky foods generally aggravate this condition; therefore, the soft, liquid diet is preferred. When the patient is being fed by tube, frequent mouth washes are desirable. In view of the well-established relationship between vitamin A and mucopolysaccharide synthesis, it might be of interest to determine whether a high vitamin A supplement can provide any additional benefit for the patient with xerostomia or mucositis.

The patient with normal masticatory function and without xerostomia should eat a detergent diet as a highly desirable aid to good oral hygiene and caries prevention. In addition, careful attention to oral hygiene, the use of topical fluorides, the mastication of fresh fruits, vegetables, and coarse fibrous foods will help prevent caries.

It would be of great interest to determine the most efficient technique or combination of techniques for self-administered topical fluoride treatment in the dying patient—including such easily controlled methods as a fluoridated mouthwash. Since the dietary composition and consistency can be regulated by the use of a blender-strained food preparation, it would also be of considerable interest to determine the effect of a noncariogenic diet in contrast to the frequently used high carbohydrate (lactose) and high calcium diets which are known to promote growth of the oral micro-organisms presumably implicated in caries.

Infection

The cause of an infection will influence the method of its treatment. An understanding of the most common situations in which infection occurs and in which treatment may lead to infection should aid in prevention and in early recognition. The most frequently observed situations in local oral pathology are:

1. Local erosion. When the skin or mucous membranes are eroded, the protection of the underlying tissues may be diminished and infection may result.

2. Lymph nodes. The natural drainage of infected tumors can lead to lymphadenitis, cellulitis, or local abscesses; the lymph nodes may contain pathogenic organisms as well as metastatic cancer. This is a common situation with intraoral cancer.

3. Necrosis. Rapidly growing neoplasms may outgrow their blood supply and the resultant central necrotic region provides an excellent culture medium. Debris from other oral lesions, i.e., periodontitis, similarly facilitates infection.

4. Lowered patient resistance. Abnormalities which affect the myeloproliferative tissues may result in sparse or abnormal leukocytes and a concomitant lowering of local resistance to infection. In addition, there may also be alterations in immune globins so that circulating antibody responses are adversely affected. Both the immune globin response and the regenerative capacity of the body are further diminished by cachexia, as well as by radiotherapy and chemotherapy. Use of systemic steroids may, through a variety of mechanisms, facilitate development of candidiasis and other local infections.

5. Factors in diagnostic procedures and treatment. It is always possible to complicate a diagnostic procedure by the introduction of infectious agents. Thus biopsies, tracheostomies, endoscopic procedures, and dental extractions may lead to infection.

When ulceration and interruption of tissue continuity are found, infection should be presumed to be present. Unfortunately, there is a paucity of research data regarding which organisms predominate in oral infections. It is clear, however, that oral monilial infections occur frequently. Also implicated are nonmonilial oral infections, staphylococci, streptococci, proteus and diphtheroid organisms.

The most common causes of systemic infections which may affect the oral care of the dying patient. are: (1) the existence of an oral infection due to the local complications outlined above, (2) debilitations and prolonged bed rest (pneumonia), (3) leukopenia secondary to antitumor chemotherapy or extensive X-irradiation, and (4) the presence of infection at some other site, not necessarily related to the oral lesion (e. g., chronic pyelonephritis).

There are no convincing data to indicate that the dying patient is inordinately susceptible to systemic bacterial infections in the absence of predisposing factors. Of more recent interest is the increasing incidence of non-bacterial infections, with yeast and fungi, or the activation of latent infections, e.g., toxoplasmosis. The apparent increase in the incidence of these infections may be related in part to the more successful management and longer survival of the dying patient. Drug therapy may impair the host's defenses and subject the patient to these apparently less commonly recognized infections.

Treatment of the systemic infection is based on the elimination of an underlying predisposing factor, as outlined above and the administration of systemic antibiotics, particularly when clinical and or microbiologic evidence of infection is clearly demonstrated. The choice of antibiotic depends on suitable microbial-sensitivity testing procedures and will also be dependent on such factors as the severity of the infection, the presence of neutropenia, the oral and general systemic status of the patient, the potential hazards relating to the development of resistant organisms, and the patient's allergic history. Gamma globulin injections (10 ml) may lessen the frequency and severity of infection, but usually will do so only for patients with hypoglobulinemia or dysproteinemia.

There is no convincing evidence that small or large doses of adrenal steroids have a beneficial effect on bacterial infections. Nevertheless, occasional patients who appear moribund do respond when treated with massive amounts of a potent glucocorticoid. It would appear reasonable to give such agents to patients who have overwhelming, life-threatening infections; to patients whose deterioration is rapid despite appropriate antimicrobials; or to patients in whom septic shock appears. A satisfactory program is the administration of 500 gm of methyl prednisolone intravenously for 24 hours per day for 3 days. The daily dose is then reduced to 250 mg on the fourth day, 125 mg on the fifth day, 60 mg on the sixth day, 30 mg on the seventh day, after which the drug is discontinued.

In instances when surgery is contemplated, preoperative prophylactic antibiotic therapy may be indicated. It is also indicated in contaminated cases, where the viability of tissues will be questionable, or a residual dead space is unavoidable. Antibiotic pretreatment or initial concomitant antibiotic treatment is favored when planning chemotherapy for oral cancer in patients with local findings which could be due to infection. Moderate doses of tetracycline, streptomycin, penicillin, or ampicillin are adequate.

The management of the febrile patient, in whom the diagnostic evaluation has failed to reveal an etiology for the fever and for whom the presumptive diagnosis is a bacterial infection, is difficult and must be resolved on the basis of that particular individual's circumstances. If the infection is presumed to be hospital-acquired, then vigorous antibacterial chemotherapy with bacteriocidal antibiotics appears warranted.

It should be stressed that vigorous therapy of infections in dying patients may be warranted because it may prolong life (where appropriate), mitigate discomfort (diaphoresis, pain, chills) and abort further deterioration of local, e.g., oral, tissues. The best control of infection is prophylaxis, and a major factor in the reduction of the frequency of oral infections in the dying patient is the improvement of oral hygiene before the patient's condition progresses to that state termed 'dying.'

Fever

Moderate elevation of body temperature does not necessarily cause discomfort, but marked elevations (above 103°) or rapid oscillations in temperature (fever spikes) can precipitate restlessness and malaise. Persistent fever may markedly enhance loss of water, requiring fluid administration to maintain the extracorpuscular fluid volume and hence allay thirst and dehydration. Antipyretic drugs, sponging with volatile solutions (usually an alcohol-water mixture), cooling mattresses, and refrigerated tents represent some of the techniques useful in the symptomatic control of fever. Attention to the precipitating cause (e.g., infection) may be more effective because the chilling effect which may accompany transitory lowering of temperature may be more unpleasant than the fever itself.

Pain

Although pain per se is not a frequent complaint of dying patients, complaints of soreness, tenderness, discomfort, and even frank pain may appear at some stage. Pain is difficult to define because there are great differences in responses to pain among patients. Furthermore, the situational psychological status of the patient (e.g., anxiety and depression) modulates the 'innate' sensitivity of the person to pain.

The causes of pain in the mouth are numerous and varied. These include: ulceration; infection; interference with mouth functions by abnormal masses (tumors, prostheses, feeding tubes); invasion of bone and nerve structures by tumors or infection; and the direct sequelae of surgical procedures, radiation therapy, and cancer chemotherapy. Pain is also a symptom associated with mouth dryness, drooling, moniliasis, and osteoradionecrosis. It should also be emphasized that in some cases pain results from the use of irritating agents such as foods and fluids, including those with an acid pH, and from the use of alcohol and tobacco. It is obvious that the dying patient is also prone to dental abnormalities (caries, odontogenic infections, defective fillings, and periodontal diseases) and that these conditions may be the sole source of pain or may intensify the symptoms emanating from the sources mentioned above. Finally, extra-oral sites may potentiate or engender pain in the oral region, e.g., the pain associated with infarction of the posterior myocardial wall may be referred to the mandibles.

The management of such symptoms as local soreness, tenderness, discomfort, and mild pain may be adequately achieved through the use of one or more of a variety of methods including: (1) application of topical protectants, denture adhesive powders and pastes, (i.e., Orahesive Bandage) for the symptomatic control of mild inflammation, erosions, and ulcerations; (2) thermal palliative approaches (ice pack, heat pad, warm saline washes) for the symptomatic control of traumatic lesions, mild infections, swellings, and edema; and (3) drugs.

The are several drug groups which may be found to be moderately effective in controlling these symptoms but their degree of effectiveness is often limited by the specific cause of the complaint.

    a. *Analgesics* (i.e., aspirin, APC, Darvon, Codeine)
    b. *Topical Anesthetics* (Xylocaine Viscous and Xylocaine ointment, benzocaine lozenges and paste, and Nupercaine lozenges)
    c. *Antimicrobial Agents* for controlling painful symptomatology associated with infection (topical and systemic antibiotics, surfactants, peroxides, and iodine formulations)
    d. *Astringents* (mouth rinses of strong tea) and mild obtundents such as Chloraseptic spray
    e. *Psychopharmacologic Agents:* antianxiety agents (Miltown, Librium, Barbiturates); antipsychotic agents (Thorazine); and antidepressants (Tofranil) for controlling longer lasting and persistent complaints wherein emotional factors are believed to be contributory
    f. *Topical Corticosteroids* (Kenalog in Orabase, various steroid

ointments) for depressing symptoms associated with the inflammation of erosions and ulcerations.

Unfortunately, despite the availability of numerous and varied approaches for controlling the mouth symptoms of the dying patient, there clearly remains a need for clinical research in this area since the results of therapy are most often less than satisfactory.

Frank Pain

The cause of frank pain should, of course, be determined before a therapeutic approach is attempted. Sometimes associated infection may be the cause of dull, constant pain. Cleaning the infection in the mouth or draining an abscess may relieve the pain more successfully than an anodyne. Constant, sharp, severe pain may be present when a tumor invades or compresses sensory nerves. Bone pain, caused by metastatic disease, may be dull or sharp; in either instance, local radiotherapy or surgical decompression may provide excellent relief. Peripheral nerve interruption may be accomplished by the injection of alcohol or an aqueous solution of five-seven per cent phenol. This is, however, a useful procedure only if the pain is localized to a small area.

It is uncommon for most patients to require potent analgesics. The demonstration of interest by the physician and his presence or ready accessibility often suffice to allay fear and pain. When drug therapy is considered, the role of such noxious agents as tobacco and alcohol in the genesis of pain should also be evaluated and attempts made to eliminate them. When analgesics are necessary, it is best to start with aspirin. The combination of aspirin and a mild sedative may be sufficient for the remainder of the patient's life. The next step is the addition of codeine to the aspirin. When stronger narcotics are required, it is best to start with small doses and use the patient's response as the indication for dosage. Phenergan or Thorazine can potentiate the effects of the narcotic agents.

Intractable Pain. When pain becomes intractable and all conservative measures have failed, peripheral neurotomy and cranial nerve section may give excellent relief of intractable oral pain. Cingulotomy and prefrontal lobotomy may change the patient's reaction to pain. These techniques are to be considered only in a minute fraction of patients who suffer from absolutely intractable pain associated with anxiety and severe emotional disturbances.

Hematologic Complications

Anemia. The anemia of the dying patient is usually mild. Although adequate statistics are not available, the most common cause of more profound anemia in the dying patient is probably a combination of acute or chronic hemorrhage, infection, and malnutrition. A specific lesion is usually the source of the bleeding, but hemorrhage may also develop from vascular abnormalities (e.g., avitaminosis), atrophy of the subcutaneous tissues, or, rarely, from coagulation defects. The latter may be related to hepatic insufficiency with failure of the protein synthesis involved in normal coagulation, e.g., hypoprothrombinemia, the *de novo* elaboration of circulating anticoagulants, or the presence of dysproteinemia in the occasional patient with a lymphoid malignancy. The infection associated with hematologic complications may be local or systemic in origin but is usually of some week's duration, since the average red cell life span is 120 days.

In the dying patient, nutritional deficiency is rarely confined to a single essential nutritional substance, but, frequently, the deficiency of one factor predominates. The patient's current state and his antecedent nutritional status must be considered to determine whether the deficiency is vitamin, mineral, or protein. Nutritional deficiency need not be related directly to the major disease but may reflect the presence of a second condition, e.g., malabsorption in a patient with terminal cancer.

Treatment with marrow-suppressive agents, such as antitumor chemotherapy or, in an occasional patient, extensive X-irradiation, may produce anemia. Furthermore, certain therapeutic agents may induce a dose-dependent anemia, e.g., phenacetin, or a sensitivity-type (glucose-6-phosphate dehydrogenase deficiency) anemia (e.g., vitamin K substitutes, sulfonamides, penicillin, streptomycin). Hemolytic episodes may occur in patients with inherited defects, such as hemoglobinopathies and enzyme deficiencies, or after blood transfusions. Acquired hemolytic states may be associated with certain neoplasms, particularly of lymphoid origin. Finally, myelophthisic anemia or leuko-erythroblastosis may develop when the marrow is invaded by tumor cells.

It is clear, then that the patient may have an anemia of complex origin resulting from: (1) impaired blood production resulting from deficiency of essential metabolites, infection, or hypoplasia induced by chemical or physical agents; (2) blood loss; (3) excessive destruction of red corpuscles; or (4) faulty construction of red cells. The exact etiology must be determined by careful diagnostic procedures and, where indicated, an attempt made to correct anemia. The decision to correct the anemia will, of course, again depend upon the total evaluation of the dying patient. The treatment of the anemia will reflect the underlying cause. Transfusion replacement with fresh blood, elimination of offending organisms or chemotherapeutics, and adequate nutrition represent the optimal treatment for anemia in the dying patient. Although androgenic substances may occasionally have a stimulatory hematopoietic effect, these agents have been found to be relatively unsatisfactory. Despite these therapeutic procedures, a mild chronic normocytic anemia may persist, usually caused by cachexia.

Leukopenia. The dying patient may have abnormalities of the leukocytes and platelets. Most commonly the leukocytes are elevated by infection and may attain leukemoid levels. Myelophthisic anemia may also produce a leukoerythroblastosis associated with the release of immature white cells. Conversely, leukopenia may reflect the presence of gram-negative infections, vigorous chemo—and radiotherapy or sensitivity to a drug. Analgesics (aminopyrine, dipyrone, phenylbutazone), procaine amide, and barbiturates have been associated with leukopenia. Cachexia itself may induce leukopenia, and specific tumors (lymphomas and leukemias) may be associated with differential inhibition of a specific cell type. Neutropenia is of importance since absolute levels below 1,500 neutrophils per cubic millimeter may predispose the patient to infection. The management of leukopenia rests primarily on the elucidation of the etiologic agent and its removal. Vigorous antibiotic therapy, judicious use of antitumor chemotherapy and X-irradiation and maintenance of nutrition are important. Infection in the presence of leukopenia is best managed by the utilization of bacteriocidal agents. White blood cell transfusion must still be considered, at present, an experimental technique.

Thrombocytopenia. The causes of thrombocytosis and thrombocytopenia in the dying patient are, in general, similar to those of leukopenia. Platelet levels may be increased and produce thromboses or be decreased and result in purpura. Thrombocytopenia may be produced by X-irradiation, antitumor chemotherapy, or other therapeutic agents. Thrombocytopenia has been noted after therapy with meprobamate, phenobarbital, sulfonamides, streptomycin, oxytetracycline, chloramphenicol, salicylates, and phenylbutazone to cite but a few agents. Platelet levels below 60,000 to 70,000 per cubic millimeter may be associated with a hemorrhagic diatheses. Again, therapy should be directed at eliminating the etiologic agent. Prednisone, approximately 30 mg per day, orally, may lessen thrombocytopenic purpura. Platelet transfusions may be used on a daily basis during severe thrombocytopenia.

The effects are temporary and antiplatelet antibodies may develop.

Paradoxically, the invasion of the marrow by neoplastic cells may require antitumor chemotherapy despite the presence of anemia, leukopenia, thrombocytopenia, and the attendant hazard of further temporary marrow hypoplasia. Under these circumstances, the attempt to eliminate the metastatic cells by use of antitumor chemotherapy should be made by a physician skilled in the administration of such agents.

Gastro-intestinal Disturbances

The patient dying from cancer, either of primary gastro-intestinal origin or metastatic to the gastro-intestinal tract and its appendages, is heir to various symptoms and physical disturbances which may affect oral hygiene. Obstruction, ileus and gastric retention may result in nausea and vomiting (as well as pain). Attention to oral hygiene may mitigate retention of debris, odors and altered taste. In the patient who has repeated episodes of vomiting, prochlorperazine, intra-muscularly, 10 mg may provide relief. This drug may precipitate extra pyramidal reactions or potentiate the pharmacologic effects of the opiates and should therefore be utilized with caution in aged patients. Chlorpromazine may not only control vomiting but potentiate the narcotic and sedative drugs. Decompressive intubation may provide relief from abdominal distension as well as vomiting, retching and air swallowing. Intubation may be irritating to the oral tissues and may restrict cough (thereby leading to atelectasis and associated complications). Alimentary tract decompression may be achieved surgically by a variety of techniques.

Cardio-pulmonary Disturbances

The dying patient may suffer from a variety of cardiac or pulmonary abnormalities which may affect his oral environment. Red cell mass, blood volume, or cardiac output may decrease to a point where insufficient oxygen transport takes place. Compensatory mechanisms of increased cardiac rate may be exceeded and restlessness from chronic anoxia occurs. Marked tachycardia can be unpleasant and tachypnea may add to terminal discomfort. Congestive heart failure may increase intra-pulmonary fluid and precipitate dyspnea. Exaggerated respiratory efforts may aggravate dryness of the mouth. Transfusion, digitalization and other supportive therapy may, therefore, contribute indirectly to oral hygiene.

The oral environment of the dying patient may be altered indirectly by a multitude of other physical and psychological factors (e.g., insomnia, decubiti, loneliness, patient-family relationships). The principle guiding the management of such a patient is universal: that which is offered to the dying patient is offered within the context of the patient as a constellation of complex inter-relations, both personal and societal. Further comfort, oral hygiene and oral function need to be evaluated on a chronological basis. A protracted demise focuses attention upon nutrition and may warrant surgical intervention. The expectation of imminent demise may preclude surgery. In the final analysis the successful care of the dying patient rests upon the physician's humility. Whereas death is relatively absolute, there are no clearly discernable or irrevocable dimensions to the dying state. The total patient is dominant.

The Radiotherapist's Relationship to the Dying Patient

Harry L. Berman*

A patient's attitude toward his malignancy and its various aspects, and the attitude of the members of his family, will involve all of the attending physicians, and this involvement ought to be one of a continuing relationship. At a time when increasing specialization in medical practice limits the attention of many physicians and surgeons to particular, localized regions of the body, terminal care has tended to become a neglected area of serious medical and social concern. It should be recognized that the dying patient presents himself as a psychosocial as well as a medical problem.

The radiological oncologist's concern and involvement, as is true for those physicians and surgeons who refer patients to him, begin with the initial consultation and meeting with the patient and the members of his family and continue throughout the course of the disease. At the outset, it will seldom be possible for the radiologist to deal with a patient on the basis of complete frankness regarding the details of the nature of his disease. The radiologist may or may not be aware of what the patient has been told in this regard by the referring physician or what the wishes of the patient's family are. The author's general rule is initially to be politely evasive until given the full information about the patient's condition and until the patient is better known to him. These factors enable the practitioner to assess the patient's reactions to what might be told him. In some instances, when the prognosis is obviously very good, no problem exists, but generally we must be concerned with patients whose prognosis is poor.

Furthermore, it may not be possible at this time to provide an explanation, giving exact details about management of the disease and its potential complications and sequelae. Essential clinical information may be lacking. An accurate prognosis may be difficult to ascertain and survival percentages are meaningless when applied to the prognosis of one patient. What is meant when a physician tells a patient that his chances for a five-year survival are 20%, or 50%, or 80%? What is unknown and unpredictable is all too frequent and pervasive. It seems reasonable for the

---

* Department of Radiation Therapy, Sinai Hospital of Baltimore, Baltimore, Maryland.

physician to offer hope to a patient, to avoid a definitive statement of a dismal prognosis, and to soften the prediction of a despairing outcome with encouraging, euphemistic phraseology—in plain words, to tell the truth but not quite the whole truth. It is not the physician's role to minimize the seriousness of a bad situation; neither should it be his mission to expose the entire appalling truth to the patient.

Informed consent will be needed for diagnostic and therapeutic procedures, the purpose of which may be quite obvious. A surgeon, advising a woman with a lump in one of her breasts to have an immediate biopsy and possible mastectomy, does not have to spell out a diagnosis. The patient knows that cancer is a possibility. Similarly, a radiologist does not lead a patient into a cobalt-60 teletherapy room for treatment, with numerous "Caution" signs prominently displayed, and then blandly tell the patient that it is treatment for a benign lesion.

While the patient has been told something less than the full truth, the radiologist's conversation with the family usually can be more candid. The need for information may be urgent so that a patient's private affairs and responsibilities can be attended to. The family in turn will likely ask some pertinent questions, such as:
1) How effective will the planned program of therapy be?
2) How much disability and suffering is to be expected?
3) Can the patient carry on normal activities?
4) How much will the treatment cost?
5) Is death imminent?
6) How long will the patient live?

Obviously, none of these questions will be easy to answer. The most that can be done is to give factual information, to admit the lack of knowledge when such is the case, and to be available for additional questions when changes in the situation occur. When the course of disease from diagnosis to death is short, the physical, psychological and economic problems facing the family may not be great. In those instances when the course of disease is protracted, all problems may be of great magnitude.

Few persons recognize cancer as anything but a serious, rapidly advancing, life-curtailing disease. Few are prepared to accept with equanimity the sudden, critical change in their pattern of living resulting from the introduction of and close association with a cancer patient in a family group. Expressed concern in the patient's disease and his progress, and emotional availability to and empathy with the patient's family on the part of his physicians are essential and rewarding requirements for the care of the cancer patient in all stages of his disease.

When an appropriate relationship with his patient has been established, the radiologist can then proceed with the evaluation of the disease, the decision about the type of therapy indicated, details of the radiation therapy plan if that modality is selected and finally, attention to specific items which may be necessary when treatment is in progress.

Head and Neck Malignancies

For the remainder of this chapter we will concern ourselves primarily with cancer of the head and neck since radiation therapy of a malignancy elsewhere in the body does not give rise to oropharyngeal symptoms. One of the first decisions to be faced by the radiologist is the determination of whether cure is possible, in which case a program of intensive, definitive therapy will be pursued even though this might involve the risk of major complications. If it is determined that cure is not likely, no purpose will be served by exposing the patient to these risks. The lesser objective of palliation directed towards improvement of the patient's comfort will then be in order.

How good are the methods to insure proper selection of patients for curative therapy? As we shall see, they leave much to be desired. There is an established system of clinical staging of head-and-neck cancers which permits surgeons and radiologists to select patients with good prognoses, to separate them from those with poor prognoses, and to apply appropriate methods of therapy for both groups. Generally, the patients with small, early lesions, localized to the sites of their origin without regional lymph node or distant metastases, have the best prognoses.

At the other extreme are those patients with far advanced stages, in which one will find the presence of massive primary tumors, large, matted, fixed masses of metastatic cervical nodes, and/or distant metastases. The recognition of the extremes is not difficult, but between them is a large intermediate group where accurate staging may not be simple and where prognosis and selection of appropriate therapy are not easily done. Under such circumstances, when the ultimate fate of the patient cannot be predicted, the tendency is to offer the patient the best chance for cure by advising him to accept the same aggressive treatment which would be indicated for the most favorable stages.

Therefore, in any given series of patients, the number of failures will be high and what is done for many patients will be in excess of actual requirements—often involving both the mutilating sequelae of radical surgery and the discomforts sequential to intensive radiation therapy. Clearly, it can be stated that too much will be done for the patient destined for an early death from his cancer and that his therapy may contribute to his discomfort, while adding nothing to his longevity. It seems that under present circumstances this situation cannot be altered, since accuracy of prognosis leaves much to be desired and current ethical principles oblige the physician to do his utmost for the patient.

To illustrate this problem, let us consider the results of treatment of carcinoma of the oral tongue according to stage at the M. D. Anderson Hospital in Houston, Texas, where surgery and radiation therapy of superb quality are available. McComb and Fletcher (1) report the results as shown in Table I.

Carcinoma of the oral tongue has been selected because this tumor lends itself readily to early recognition and is accessible for treatment by surgery or radiation therapy or a combination of both. As can be seen in Table I, the majority of the patients came to the hospital in an early stage (Stages I and II). These patients experienced discomfort early and could recognize the presence of their tumor. It is in this group that the greatest percentage of survivors for five or more years is found. Nevertheless, we note that:

1) while the five-year survival rate is 50%, the five-year failure rate is also 50%;
2) a large number of patients died of causes other than cancer
3) the remaining number of deaths was caused by persistent, recurrent or metastatic malignant disease (17 of 103 patients).

In the group of advanced cancer patients (Stages III and IV) those surviving free of disease comprised 16 of 73. As might be expected, the number dying of uncured malignant disease was predominantly high (46 of 73), while those dying of intermittent diseases other than cancer comprised 11 of 73. It seems obvious that the reason for the last figure is the fact that most members of this group died of their malignancy, even though some might have had serious intercurrent diseases from which they might have died, if they survived long enough after effective treatment of their cancers. We have considered the results of therapy under the best circumstances for one of the less fatal types of head and neck cancers. In others types of cancers, such as the cancers of the nasopharynx, the outlook is even gloomier.

TABLE I

Stage	No. Pts.	Died of Disease	Died of Other Causes	Alive N E D
I	53	6	16	29
II	50	11	15	23
III	31	16	6	9
IV	42	30	5	6
Totals	176	63	42	67

While these facts indicate that much of what is done in the name of definitive cancer therapy represents a prodigious effort involving considerable professional skill and great expense and culminates too often in end results that are far from gratifying, it is still doubtful that this situation can be readily changed. Even with greater accuracy in staging and improvement in the selection of patients for appropriate therapy, the parameters of a given tumor related to degree of malignancy, propensity for its dissemination, the host reaction and its capacity for limiting tumor spread remain unknown and impossible to measure.

Careful staging does not insure the examiner that microsopic deposits of tumor have not been overlooked; and all modalities of therapy, no matter how carefully and methodically performed, have an indeterminate measure of geographic misses. Furthermore, whatever elements of carcinogenesis might be present in a specific patient, ablation of his tumor will not necessarily result in their elimination. It is readily apparent that terminal care will be the certain fate of a great number of patients with head-and-neck cancer, and that this will occur even though we understand that a large number of patients will be treated energetically to salvage the relatively small number we do.

Nevertheless, we should keep trying to improve our staging procedures to insure a better selection of patients for curative therapy, and for a more critical examination of patients for the presence of intercurrent diseases likely to produce early mortality. When the chances for success are pitifully low, one must question whether a radical procedure represents a real accomplishment in view of the mutilation of extensive surgery, the uncomfortable consequences of intensive, high-dose irradiation, and the severe, debilitating effects of some of our current chemotherapy.

Fundamental radio-biology in clinical use, the combined use of surgery and pre-operative irradiation, and the joint administration of chemotherapy with radiation therapy are being investigated. All pose special problems in the oropharynx, since they involve the question of tolerance of normal tissues and mucosal reactions. Although radiation therapy is indicated for the definitive care of tumors in surgically inaccessible areas, it can also be used advantageously in the areas of the head and neck where surgery has its clearest indications and where competition as to choice of treatment exists. Radiation therapy is indicated especially in advanced stages in these areas when surgery is contraindicated, or when certain medical conditions make surgery undesirable.

A. B. is a 48-year-old, single, Caucasian woman who lives alone. An aged mother, living elsewhere, is her only relative. The patient was seen in consultation for an opinion regarding the management of a squamous cell carcinoma of the anterior floor of the mouth and a squamous cell carcinoma of the left ary-epiglottic fold and pyriform sinus.

The patient's daily routine includes the intake of one-tenth to one-fifth of a gallon of whiskey and smoking three packs of cigarettes. It is generally agreed that these agents play causative roles in the genesis of cancer of the oral cavity and pharynx. Abstinence from both, henceforth, will be mandatory for her. The management of either tumor poses problems of great magnitude for a normally adjusted person supported by the assistance and encouragement of relatives. The combination of the two tumors in this individual is a formidable problem of overwhelming dimensions. The cancer of the floor of the mouth, although somewhat advanced (Stage III), is potentially curable. The hypopharyngeal cancer is probably incurable. Although the patient had sought medical attention early in the course of her disease, the diagnosis was missed and its establishment was unfortunately delayed.

At this point an objective appraisal of methods of therapy under consideration included the following treatment plan:

1) removal of teeth which were not in good condition;
2) radiation therapy of both lesions;
3) radium implant for the mouth lesion followed by bilateral suprahyoid neck dissection and total laryngectomy;
4) commando resection of the mouth lesion and bilateral suprahyoid neck dissection, and external irradiation for the hypopharyngeal tumor.

The management of her problem was discussed with the patient in reasonably softened and general terms, but she had little doubt that she was confronted by a terrible predicament and that considerable disfigurement and mutilation would be the result of her surgery. She chose no treatment. The author did not see her again. Since spontaneous regression of tumors is not an alternative on which one can rely with confidence, it seems certain that she would soon go to someone for palliative therapy. In the author's opinion she was incurable when he saw her initially. Palliative irradiation was all that was indicated; surgery should not have been suggested for her, and arrangements for her terminal care should have been made at an early date.

A 75-year-old Caucasian man was in generally good health but suffering from the mental deterioration of arteriosclerotic brain disease. He was first seen by the author in 1969 with a pyriform sinus carcinoma. He was treated with cobalt-60 teletherapy with great difficulty because of his poor cooperation. Nevertheless he fared well and the tumor was destroyed. About a year later he returned with a new carcinoma of the left lower gingiva. In order to avoid the difficulties of trying to gain his cooperation for external beam radiation therapy, it was decided to treat him with the insertion of radon seeds under local anesthesia. Again, the tumor was successfully destroyed, but six months later he returned with a third tumor in the mucosa of the hard palate. This was successfully treated with cryosurgery. Three months after his last treatment he returned with metastatic cervical nodes. At present the treatment plan involves radon seeds. All of his treatments were palliative in intent and were conducted with a minimum of discomfort and requirement for hospitalization. Such a favorable outcome of the treatment was not anticipated. He remains disoriented and confused and we are undecided as to whether we should continue our efforts to save him.

The various aspects of head-and-neck cancer as they concern the therapeutic radiologist have been discussed, particularly in relation to the problems of terminal care. Emphasis has been placed on the fact that the radiotherapist's role should not be confined to the technical details of his modality; that his interest in the question of terminal care may be warranted at an early date; and that his treatments require a high degree of individualization. Stress was also placed on the need for better selection of patients for aggressive, definitive cancer therapy, so that patients with advanced disease will not be subjected to the severe demands of that type of treatment.

Reference

1. W. S. McComb and G. H. Fletcher, *Cancer of the Head and Neck*, Baltimore:The Williams and Wilkins Co., 1967, p. 122.

Oral Care of the Dying Patient: Neurological Aspects

Thomas J. Bridges, Jr. *

Altered neurological function may add to the usual difficulties in providing oral care for the dying patient. Neurological abnormality may require care of two types:
1) life-saving or interventive care
2) terminal (often prolonged) care.

Coma

Coma is a most common neurological state and is encountered in the most diverse group of severely ill patients. It may be encountered as an acute condition resulting from injury in young, previously healthy persons, or as a chronic condition in terminally ill patients dying of cancer or neurological disease. It may be reversible, fluctuating, progressive or static.

Oral care for the comatose patient may be life-saving or essential to life support. The patient's needs are:
1) maintenance of the airway
2) removal of secretions
3) substitution of other routes of supply of fluids and food.

When coma is of rapid onset and deep, respiratory inadequacy is a real threat to life. Insertion of an endotracheal tube prevents the tongue from blocking the oropharyngeal airway, the flaccid pharyngeal and laryngeal muscles are bypassed and even weak or irregular diaphragmatic-thoracic muscular activity can maintain an adequate intake of oxygen (air) and expulsion of carbon dioxide. In the event of inadequate diaphragmatic function, respiratory assistance may be added via the endotracheal tube by the use of an external ventilation machine operating on demand or by self-regulation.

Secretions require attention and may be aspirated. Secretions which collect in the mouth are most easily removed by placing the patient in a position to permit continuous drainage from the mouth. When it is not possible to utilize position to effect drainage, oral suction is required. Although this method is effective, it requires the help of a nurse or

---
* Neurological Institute, Columbia-Presbyterian Medical Center, New York, New York.

attendant; it is intermittent, and the indication for suction can be detected or signaled only by a companion of the patient. Continuous, low pressure oral suction tends to become ineffective due to the malplacement of the suction tip, change in position in relation to the pool of secretions, or by plugging of the tubing.

Fluid support is essential to avoid dehydration in those comatose patients for whom there is hope for survival and for patients in prolonged coma. In the early stages of coma, intravenously administered fluids are satisfactory. Transfusion, when indicated, implies the intravenous route. After about three days, other routes of fluid supply should be sought. The most frequently used route for long-term fluid support is nasogastric.

There are limitations on the types of fluids which may be administered intravenously, compared with those which may be supplied by gastric tube. High caloric formula, containing a broader range of minerals and vitamins, are usually available to the tube-fed patient. It is recognized that gastric absorption may well occur at a rate best suited to the patient's need. It is sometimes forgotten that a broad range of medication, such as analgesics, laxatives or anticonvulsants, may be readily given by gastric tube. This technique of administration allows not only the use of a broad range of medication but gradual absorption, and a lessened risk of needle-site infection as well.

Orogastric tube feeding may be utilized if the nasal route is not available, or in long-term cases, as an intermittent alternate. Rectally administered fluid may be absorbed, but the volume rate of absorption is not predictable. When the oral route is not feasible, gastrostomy may permit the administration of fluids and of food.

The problems of the neurological aspects of the oral care of the dying patient may be considered to have been outlined, using the comatose patient as the model. But what of the not-so-comatose patient?

Semicoma

Alterations of consciousness vary from mental dullness to deep coma. With a lesser degree of altered consciousness, the hope is that the patient should be able to assist in his own oral care. Unfortunately, lightened consciousness will at times be accompanied by irrationality, resistance to proffered assistance, irritability, or withdrawal. Behavior may vary in type over a period of time. Indeed it is easier to outline, order, and carry out a plan for provision of the oral care needed for comatose patients, than for the non-comatose group, though the same basic requirements for maintenance of respiratory function, removal of secretions, and provision of adequate food and fluids remain mandatory. The problems of oral care may be compounded notably by impaired consciousness, but also may be increased by lack of patient cooperation when a neurological deficit such as deafness, blindness, aphasia or hemiplegia exists. Dysphagia due to cranial nerve disorder or to oropharyngeal obstruction complicates the problems of oral care, as there may well be excessive salivation in the presence of difficulty in swallowing. Facial disfiguration has a profound effect on some patients, leading to depression and withdrawal from others (as well as the withdrawal of others from the patient).

A list of conditions of neurological dysfunction which may afflict dying patients and complicate oral care would be long and variable. The most common disease states of terminally ill patients are cancer and neurological diseases. The involvement varies from the neurological involvement of nervous system trauma, caused by the cerebral metastases of cancer or demylinating disease, to the aphasia and hemiphagia of cerebrovascular disease.

A glance at the range of variability of the oral needs of terminally ill patients leads to the conclusion that flexibility in systems of oral care will be required. Oral care needs will be met best by recognition of the particular needs of each case; individualization is required and, at times, improvisation in the implementation of necessary care.

Sedations or tranquilizers may be given to produce a degree of calmness and acceptance of needed care by the irrational, lethargic, uncooperative, confused or resistant patient. It is imperative that great caution and much attention be given to the administration of drugs. For example, resistance to proffered care may be due to pain on swallowing, and sedations may be ineffective whereas an analgesic might be of help.

Sedations may increase confusion or irrationality. One irrational, uncooperative head injury patient became cooperative and progressively more rational after discontinuation of sedative medication. Indeed, he had been transferred from another hospital where increasing rambunctiousness had been handled with increasing doses of sedative drugs. Elimination of sedative medication restored him to a more tractable condition.

Before attempting to modify patient behavior by drug therapy, it is essential to learn what may underlie the behavior; what the patient's previous reaction to the contemplated drug has been; and to set up with a degree of caution some method of evaluating the effect of a drug to be prescribed.

Position

Patients who are unable to cooperate fully in postural drainage therapy may resist the required position or may constantly deviate from it. Hemiplegic patients seem to favor one or the other side and usually avoid lying on the "normal" side since this limits functioning of the normal extremities.

While the three-quarter prone or lateral recumbent position may promote mouth drainage or escape of vomitus, it may be undesirable because it may limit respiratory chest motion or it may not reduce intracranial vascular tension as much as a sitting position. In prescribing patient position, one must keep in mind the primary goal, the early return of consciousness, rather than prevention of a possible complication. The primary need must be the primary determinant in the medical care of the individual patient.

Airways

Nasopharyngeal airway or endotracheal tubes are ideal because of availability and ease of insertion in acute cases requiring respiratory assistance. They are poorly tolerated in completely conscious patients and tend to produce local irritation and swallowing if left too long in place.

Tracheostomy is better tolerated by the conscious patient and can be tolerated for prolonged periods. The "routine" use of tracheostomy after the removal of large accoustineurinoma tumors has resulted in a marked decrease in morbidity and mortality. Tracheal suction is easily carried out. Cough is unobstructed. Valve-type closure permits vocalization earlier than with the unobstructed tracheostomy, and yet the tracheo-bronchial tree is accessible for aspiration whenever this is necessary.

When disease has obstructed the oral pharynx or larynx, tracheostomy with a plastic tracheostomy tube or surgical opening are valuable. Because tracheostomy access to the lungs permits the use of a respirator, either demand or self-regulating, it is possible to maintain the vital functions for prolonged periods of time. The physician must base his decision to prolong or terminate this "life" upon consideration of the patient and his family's real needs and desires.

Parenteral Feeding

The comatose patient will tolerate intravenous or nasogastric feedings; the not-so-comatose patient may "pull the tubes out." In cases where patient cooperation is poor, the best solution to fluid and food problems is to apply them for short periods of time. Patients may be restrained for two or four hours during the day, given intravenous or tube feedings, released, and the process repeated as needed. This requires more time and effort than a program of constant restraint, but avoids complications associated with a limited, restrained position. Large amounts of food and fluid may be given in a two-to-four hour period by gastric tube.

The drawback to the use of gastric feeding, by tube or gastrostomy, is that pleasurable experiences of eating and drinking, with their elements of taste and of touch and fullness in the mouth, are important. The conscious patient, though well hydrated and maintaining weight, finds a great sense of loss in the absence of eating, though he is being well maintained by a gastrostomy. One patient had an engineer brother devise a funnel tube device for his gastrostomy so that he might chew his food prior to its passage into the stomach through the funnel and tube.

Facial palsy may cause the escape of liquids and occasionally food from the corner of the mouth on the side of the facial paralysis. This may be reduced to some degree by external skin strapping to elevate the corner of the mouth. In chronic cases, the use of internal (subcutaneous) facial slings or re-innervation by nerve suture or nerve transplant may be most helpful.

When 7th and 5th nerve palsies occur together, swallowing is more difficult because of loss of sensation within the mouth (and tongue) on the side of the trigeminal nerve lesion. Patients who can place food in the normally innervated side of the mouth can eat more easily. This point should be known to aids who help spoon-feed patients.

Glossopharyngeal-vagal swallowing deficits manifest themselves by choking upon swallowing effort. Initially, these patients require parenteral feeding. When the patient can draw liquid into the mouth through a straw, he is ready to try swallowing. Soft, semi-solid food, such as baby food, is more easily tolerated than are fluids. In cases of pharyngeal or laryngeal lesion, swallowing may be extremely painful. Analgesics may be helpful. Surgical section of the appropriate cranial nerves may be a very valuable procedure though it is limited in application to patients well enough to undergo a cranial operation and whose expectancy is such as to make the operation worthwhile.

Paralysis of one hypoglossal nerve is well tolerated. Bilateral hypoglossal palsy with paralysis of the tongue leads to the threat of asphyxiation by the backward going tongue, and to marked difficulty with verbalization and with chewing. Such patients eat with difficulty and will require supplemental or total parenteral administration of food and fluid.

Pseudo-bulbar effects of cerebral disease, such as stroke or neoplasm, result in loss of voluntary control of muscles of the oral and pharyngeal cavities and larynx. This interferes with speech and leads to the deep "gutteral" voice. There is difficulty with swallowing fluids or solids. Oral care is similar to that required for lesions of the mouth and 9th and 10th cranial nerves. (In addition, these patients may exhibit organically-determined emotional changes, as well as psychic reaction to their illness in the form of depression with loss of appetite and withdrawal.)

Facial prosthesis to obtain separation of oral from sinus cavities, or oral cavity from the external or skin area, may again allow the patient to eat, talk and breathe better.

The above considerations involve what can be done to the patient for his advantage. A last consideration is what can be done in the way of oral care to the patient for the advantage of those around him.

Death should come graciously for the patient. It is gratifying when it also comes graciously for his relatives, for his friends, for those who care for him.

Disfigurement results from disease and from treatment. The patient knows that his individuality is in his face and the structures behind it. It is sad when treatment fails and death is ensuing; doubly sad when treatment leads to an appearance which is revolting to those who are close to the patient and who will remember him after his death.

It is not enough to supply fluid and food to the ill. It is imperative that everything possible be done to help the terminal patient continue to live as the individual he is, and, if his appearance is changed, either by disease or treatment, that the crutch or the make-up needed to maintain the patient's basic individuality be provided.

Bibliography

J. C. Quint, "Nursing Care of the Terminal Patient," chapter in B. Schoenberg, A. C. Carr, D. Peretz and A. H. Kutscher (Eds.), *Psychosocial Aspects of Terminal Care*, New York: Columbia University Press, 1972.

Cancer Chemotherapy: Implications for the Dentist

*Susan Mellette**

Only a few years ago, the patient with malignant disease which had continued to spread after surgery or radiation therapy could be offered no specific treatment. Then followed a decade or two during which cytotoxic chemical agents came into use in a relatively small number of medical centers. Currently, over twenty antitumor agents of the cytotoxic types are commercially available. Many patients are treated on an ambulatory basis; and many physicians with relatively little experience or training in the use of these chemicals are administering them to their patients. More and more patients who are receiving one or another of the cancer chemotherapeutic agents will be presenting themselves to their dentists, either for unrelated dental problems or, not infrequently, for oral complaints which may be the direct result of their anti-tumor treatment. The dentist today has to have some basic knowledge about cancer chemotherapy: what these agents are, how well they work, and how their side effects may influence his own decisions in regard to dental procedures or oral care.

Undue concern about the medication being given may be transmitted to the patient who usually needs reassurance rather than uncertainty. Usually, it is the physician or dentist who is unfamiliar with current cancer chemotherapy who, sometimes inadvertently, leaves his patient feeling that he, himself, is frightened by "those poisons" the patient is receiving. In any case, a close working relationship between the medical oncologist or other physician who has prescribed the chemotherapeutic agent and the patient's dentist is highly desirable and sometimes essential to the patient's best interests. Such a cooperative endeavor is optimal when the dentist already has a general fund of information about cancer chemotherapy, particularly as it may affect his own field.

Mechanism of Action of Antitumor Agents

No drugs have as yet been found which are specifically lethal only to cancer cells. In general, however, the drugs found useful in cancer

---

* Medical College of Virginia, Richmond, Virginia.

chemotherapy are capable of producing greater damage to neoplastic cells than to normal cells, presumably because of metabolic differences between these cells. Recently, it has become apparent that the actual rate of cell division is not as important a difference as was formerly supposed; but less well-defined biochemical characteristics of the cancer cell may be quantitatively sufficiently unlike those of normal cells to allow for some relative selectivity of cellular damage. The particular type of cancer cell involved is a major determining factor in the selection of an agent. For example, a cancer with its origin in the gastrointestinal tract is ordinarily untouched by clinically usable doses of agents which will produce marked shrinkage or destruction of the enlarged nodes of lymphosarcoma. Conversely, doses of the antimetabolic agent which can yield marked improvement in the patient with colon cancer have little or no effect on a lymphosarcoma. To some degree, at least, we are not operating in a hit-and-miss manner in cancer chemotherapy, although most of the available information was achieved originally only by clinical trials in consenting patients. Furthermore, as the agents differ in their effects on cancer cells so do the side effects or the concurrent damage induced in normal body cells.

Cancer chemotherapeutic agents are generally grouped according to their mode of action at the cellular level or their source or general chemical type. These classifications are of some convenience although it is recognized that, for at least some agents, more than one type of action may occur. Since cellular function and replication are basically dependent on continuing synthesis of DNA, it is not unexpected that most of the cancer chemotherapeutic agents act at some point which involves DNA.

1. *Alkylating agents,* including the "prototype antitumor agent" nitrogen mustard and some related compounds, act by the substitution of an alkyl group on a reactive site. Cross-linking of strands of DNA or selective reaction with guanine to break a strand may occur. Both resting and proliferating cells may be injured in a relatively non-specific fashion similar to that of irradiation—an effect which has resulted in these compounds often being called "radiomimetic agents." Current information indicates that some of the agents generally included in this group, e.g., cyclophosphamide, may be highly "phase-specific," that is, much more toxic to cells in the proliferative stage of their cycle. All of the agents in this group are potentially highly toxic to the hematopoietic system and this situation is complicated by the fact that they may differ in the time at which the greatest decrease in leucocyte or platelet count occurs and in the time required for recovery of the blood cells.

2. *Antimetabolites* —Such agents, through a variety of mechanisms, ultimately block DNA synthesis because of their chemical similarity to essential substances in the biosynthetic chain through which purines or pyrimidines are involved in the formation of DNA. For convenience again, these have been generally grouped as folic acid antagonists (methotrexate), purine antagonists (6-mercaptopurine) and anti-pyrimidines such as 5-fluorouracil or arabinosylcytosine. Such groupings are oversimplifications since these agents may act at more than one point. For example, methotrexate blocks folic reductase to prevent the availability of single carbon fragments needed for purine ring biosynthesis and also inhibits the methylation of deoxyuridylic acid to thymidylic acid—an essential component of DNA. From the standpoint of the dentist, however, the group of antimetabolites should be remembered as the more likely culprits in the patient developing oral ulcerations as a concomitant of antitumor therapy.

3. *Antitumor antibiotics* such as Actinomycin D, produce their effects directly on DNA—for example, by binding to DNA in such a manner that DNA dependent RNA synthesis is inhibited. In dose regimes in clinical use, such agents may produce hematopoietic, oral and gastrointestinal toxicity.

4. *Plant alkaloids*—Another variety of action on the cell is demonstrated by derivatives of Vinca rosea, a type of periwinkle plant. The agents act on the mitotic spindle to disrupt it and arrest cell division.

5. *Miscellaneous*—Some of the chemotherapeutic agents in current use do not fit particularly well into any of the above categories. One of these is Methylhydrazine (Matulane) which acts by depolymerizing DNA.

6. *Hormones*—When tissues which are sensitive to hormones are the source of the malignancy, some of the longest lasting control of metastatic malignant disease is achieved. The hormones may act on the supply of stimulating hormones of pituitary origin but it appears more and more likely that more direct effects also occur on the cancer cell. It has been postulated that this involves the protein synthetic processes, probably beyond the RNA level.

Types of Malignancy Amenable to Chemotherapy

The oral surgeon will be most commonly concerned with the

squamous cell epitheliomas arising in and around the oral cavity. Unfortunately, most of these malignancies are less responsive to presently available chemotherapeutic agents than are tumors arising in other body areas. A bit of general information as to the results currently to be expected from optimal chemotherapy is, however, useful as a part of the store of medical knowledge of the dentist. Tumors in which chemotherapy may be of significant value include:

1. Chorioepithelioma—A rare tumor arising in women from placental tissue after pregnancy, it is a highly fatal malignancy after dissemination has occurred. It may be cured in a high percentage of cases by drugs alone.

2. Childhood tumors such as Wilms tumor of the kidney and Burkitt's lymphoma also have been cured, apparently in some cases, by chemotherapy.

3. Leukemias, lymphomas including Hodgkin's disease, multiple myeloma—Definite clinical benefit and control of disease may often be achieved for months or years.

4. Carcinoma primary in breast, prostate, thyroid—When appropriately treated by hormonal agent, it may regress to apparent clinical disappearance for months to years, with subsequent regressions caused by other hormones to which the tumor cells may be sensitive, or if the administered hormone suppresses a stimulating hormone.

5. Carcinoma primary in the ovary, gastrointestinal tract, lung, and various other sites may respond with regression to appropriate chemotherapy. The degree and duration of benefit are highly variable.

6. Sarcomas, melanomas, and related tumors occasionally regress but the results obtained are often of little clinical significance.

Side Effects of Cancer Chemotherapeutic Agents of Particular Importance to the Dentist

1. *Cytopenia*—With the exception of Vincristine and, of course, the hormones, all of the antitumor agents in current use may produce a significant decrease in circulating blood cells. The cells most affected are leucocytes and platelets.

2. *Stomatitis*—The development of small ulcers of the oral mucosa, tongue or lips is a common result of treatment, particularly with the antimetabolites. In practice it has sometimes been the custom to use the development of stomatitis as an end point for deciding that optimal treatment has been given. The patient is instructed to continue taking the medication (for example, methotrexate) until ulcers develop. The ulceration is essentially indistinguishable clinically from that of herpes simplex stomatitis. It usually subsides within a day or two after the cytotoxic is discontinued. Ordinarily no specific treatment is instituted for the stomatitis; warm saline or 20% Karo mouth washes may be soothing.

3. *Neurotoxicity*—One of the most interesting and confusing of side effects which may come to the attention of the dentist is the pain in the jaw which sometimes follows the administration of Vincristine. This plant alkaloid is frequently employed alone or in combination for lymphomas, childhood tumors, and some of the soft tissue tumors. Its toxicity is primarily neurological, usually manifest by numbness and tingling in the fingers or toes after the injections have been given for several weeks and associated with loss of deep tendon reflexes in the legs. In a small number of patients, however, as noted by us and reported by others, there has been an almost immediate effect (within a day or two) in which there is pain over the parotid area and jaw, sometimes in the throat. This has subsided spontaneously.

Some Illustrative Oral Problems in Patients Receiving Antitumor Agents

J. M., a 36-year-old male, had been under treatment for three years, first with radiotherapy, then with multiple varieties of chemotherapy for Hodgkin's disease. No lymphadenopathy was detectable nor any physical evidence of activity of his Hodgkin's disease. However, he again became febrile and developed a significantly elevated sedimentation rate. Further questioning revealed that he "had been having trouble with an abscessed tooth"; and examination showed extensive purulent periodontal disease. The cancer chemotherapeutic agent was discontinued and antibacterial antibiotics given for several days followed by extraction of all remaining teeth. Blood leucocyte count had been in the 5-6,000 range just prior to the extractions but declined to less than 3,000—in spite of the fact that no further cytotoxics had been given. The interpretation of this was that the 5-6,000 count represented the maximal response which the long-suppressed bone marrow could make to the presence of infection and that his actual count in the absence of a source of stimulation was in the leukopenic range. Healing was, however, quite satisfactory and he became afebrile again. In this case, concurrent oral disease confused the interpretation both of the degree of activity of his Hodkin's disease and of his white blood cell count. If it had been assumed that he had reactivation of his Hodgkin's disease as the source of his fever and elevated sedimentation rate, he might have been given more aggressive antitumor chemotherapy which was not only unnecessary but would have further complicated the treatment of his oral problems.

H. P., a 39-year-old man with an aggressive lung cancer with multiple bony metastases, had been receiving large doses of alkylating agents and corticoids for hypercalcemia, and broad-spectrum antibiotics for the pneumonitis which is a frequent result of areas of atelectasis secondary to pulmonary neoplastic lessions. He complained bitterly one night of a sore throat. He was afebrile and had a moderate leukopenia. Examination revealed that not only the pharynx but practically the entire oral mucosa was covered with white placques, characteristic of monilial infection. The response to Mycostatin oral suspension was dramatic and he was asymptomatic within 24 hours. In this case, the patient had multiple factors contributing to his susceptibility to yeast overgrowth and debility secondary to his tumor plus treatment with adrenal hormones, cytotoxics and antibiotics.

Summary

Cancer chemotherapy has reached a level of use and recognition in which a large percentage of patients with disseminated malignancy may be receiving one or another agent or combinations of several drugs. Actual cure of metastatic choriocarcinoma, some cases of Burkitt's lymphoma, and an occasional apparent cure of a few other tumors, has been achieved by the use of antitumor chemicals alone. Types of agents in common use include alkylating agents, antimetabolites, some antitumor antibiotics, and plant alkaloids which induce mitotic arrest. Appropriate use of adrenal or gonadal hormones is also often worthwhile.

The dentist particularly needs to know some of the side effects of the cancer chemotherapeutic agents in order that he may properly care for and evaluate oral problems in patients being treated with these agents. Leucopenia and thrombocytopenia may limit the oral surgeon in performing needed procedures. The stomatitis which develops as a result of the antimetabolites or antitumor antibiotics may send the patient to his dentist rather than back to his physician. The development of pain in the jaw, following treatment with one of the neurotoxic plant alkaloids, is a side effect only recently recognized, and one for which the dentist may be first consulted.

Patients receiving antitumor agents may also have an increased susceptibility to oral moniliasis with its clinical manifestations. Resistance to other infectious processes involving the mouth may also be lowered; and the importance of good oral hygiene in these patients cannot be overemphasized.

Psychopharmacological Agents, Narcotic Analgesics and Oral Problems of the Dying Patient

Edward H. Montgomery[†] and Fred F. Cowan[*]

There is an erroneous assumption that a "dying" patient may be defined only as: a patient whose physician has officially diagnosed his present condition as terminal, and a patient who will be dead within a few hours or within a few days at the most. There are "dying" patients, however, who can and do live for a number of months or longer after such a diagnosis. In these cases the quality of oral care can play a significant role in the dying patient's comfort and waning well-being. It is not unlikely at all that such a patient will have the need for the dental practitioner's services.

It is, furthermore, not unlikely that such a patient will be taking at this time one or more psychopharmacological agents or narcotic analgesics under the supervision of the physician. Thus, the proper dental treatment of the dying patient who is concurrently taking these drugs is of considerable importance.

The dying patient may also urgently require a dentist's services on an emergency basis due to traumatic injury to the oro-facial area as a direct or indirect result of his condition. In such a situation, it is probable that the dentist may wish to administer or prescribe a narcotic analgesic to relieve severe oral pain or an anxiolytic sedative to allay apprehension.

In either case, a thorough understanding of the clinical pharmacology of these drugs is mandatory, and total cooperation between the attending physician and the dental practitioner is essential. It is not our purpose in this paper to present the pharmacologic knowledge prerequisite to such a thorough understanding; but rather to review briefly the pharmacology of several groups of psychopharmacological agents and the narcotic analgesics with emphasis on their side effects, particularly those related to oral disease and its treatment.

[†] Department of Pharmacology, University of Texas Dental School, Houston, Texas.
[*] Department of Pharmacology, University of Oregon Dental School, Portland, Oregon

I. Psychopharmacological Agents

Although the use of drugs affecting mental activity may be traced to early civilizations, it was not until the mid 1950's that chemical substances began to be used widely in the treatment of psychiatric disorders. The discovery of the beneficial effect of chlorpromazine in treating the symptoms of schizophrenia and other agitated psychotic states initiated a new era in the treatment of mental illness and gave rise to a new specialty of pharmacology, psychopharmacology (1). Psychopharmacological agents may be defined broadly as drugs which have a predominant effect on emotion, mood, perception, thinking and general behavior. These agents exert their major pharmacological effects through an action on subcortical areas of the central nervous system with a minimum of activity on the cerebral cortex. Although these agents do not cure psychiatric disorders, their introduction into psychiatry has resulted in a complete revolution in the treatment of mental illness. During the past fifteen years the number of agents conforming to this general definition has increased significantly. Their prominent place in the present therapeutic armamentarium is indicated by the fact that one-third of all outpatient prescriptions written in the United States since 1965 have been for some type of psychopharmacological agent.

The psychopharmacological agents may be categorized on the basis of their clinical usefulness into the following five subclasses: neuroleptic agents, anxiolytic sedatives, antidepressants, psychostimulants and psychodysleptics. The profound effects of these agents on behavior and emotional symptoms of certain mental diseases are accompanied by a large number of neurological side effects and other untoward reactions which apparently parallel their degree of activity on psychological and emotional processes. For example, the neuroleptic tranquilizers are not only much more effective in controlling psychological processes than are the anxiolytic tranquilizers but also are associated with a greater incidence of severe adverse reactions. Many of the numerous side effects produced by these agents are of significance in the diagnosis of oral problems and are manifested in the oro-facial region of the body. All too frequently these orally-related side effects progress either unnoticed or untreated until the patient's oral health and comfort are severely compromised.

The rationale for the use of any one or more of the psychopharmacological agents in the dying patient is as varied as the terminal illness itself. Perhaps the drug is a phenothiazine neuroleptic agent used for its antiemetic effect following X-ray therapy; or it may be an anxiolytic sedative used in the treatment of severe anxiety; or an antidepressant used in the treatment of the symptoms of senile depression. The drug may be an anxiolytic sedative such as diazepam which is being used by the dental practitioner for both its antianxiety and skeletal muscle relaxant effects in the treatment of muscle spasms associated with a temporomandibular joint disorder. The reasons for which the psychopharmacological agents are used in the dying patient are seldom unique, but major disparities in the effects produced by these agents occur as a result of the severely debilitated condition of these patients. Their use in a physically debilitated patient is associated with an increasing array and incidence of side effects of increasing severity as the patient's debilitation progresses. Whereas the xerostomia produced by chlorpromazine may be tolerated in the patient with normal defense mechanisms, this same side effect may result in a severe oral infection in the terminal cancer patient who concurrently is taking antineoplastic agents or other immunosuppressants. Furthermore, treatment of many terminal diseases requires the use of a number of drugs, many of which exhibit severe toxic reactions and side effects, e.g., cytotoxic agents in terminal cancer. In these cases, drug-drug and/or drug-disease interactions may occur with alarming frequency and severity.

In most patients the psychological trauma of approaching death is associated with anxiety, apprehension and depression. These psychological disturbances may be manifested as psychosomatic pain in the oro-facial region, dry mouth, and other symptoms of oral disease such as facial muscle spasms. It is the problem of the diagnosing practitioner to determine which symptoms are related to existent oral pathology and which are of psychological origin. In any case, the use of the usual psychopharmacological agents in treating the anxiety and/or depression of these patients would increase the severity of the existing xerostomia; oro-facial pain and other symptoms of oral disease may be increased as a result of the side effects of these drugs and not because of existent oral diseases. However, these symptoms also could be the resultant signs of drug-induced oral pathology.

Even if the disease is terminal and its treatment beyond the realm of modern medicine, it is possible to alleviate many of the patient's distressing symptoms and reduce his mental anguish to a certain degree. Concomitant oral disease not only contributes to the patient's distress and anguish but also may be a primary factor in causing his pain, suffering and anxiety. Therefore, it is the responsibility of the dentist as well as of the physician to provide the patient with the greatest degree of comfort possible. Although the patient cannot be cured of his terminal illness, oral infection or a drug-induced dystonic syndrome may be relieved adequately or eliminated.

The following discussion should not be misconstrued as an indication for the use of the *neuroleptic agents* or *antidepressant drugs* in the practice of dentistry. These agents are useful in the treatment of symptoms of severe psychiatric disorders but they are of doubtful effectiveness in neurotic conditions. The numerous side effects and adverse reactions produced by these agents preclude their use by all but the most experienced practitioners. It is because of their many side effects, some of which are manifested orally, that these agents are of significance to the dental practitioner who is asked to care for the patient's oral disease. The success of the oral treatment will depend on his knowledge of the pharmacology of these agents and his awareness of the side effects produced by these drugs. The anxious, apprehensive dental patient can be adequately controlled with agents such as the anxiolytic sedatives or barbiturates; neuroleptic drugs are not only ineffective in such conditions but also may enhance more severe psychological disturbances. The dental practitioner must realize that in the patient with terminal illness the combination of impairment of normal physiological mechanisms and drug-induced side effects not only greatly increases the risk of dental treatment but also may be the cause of the oral disease.

A. Neuroleptic Agents

As indicated by their classification, these drugs produce a type of behavioral state known as the neuroleptic syndrome. They are used clinically for their effectiveness in the control of agitation, delusions, hallucinations and other symptoms of acute or chronic agitated psychoses such as schizophrenia, mania and delirious states. The chemical classes of drugs which are used clinically as neuroleptic tranquilizers are the phenothiazine, thioxanthene and butyrophenone derivatives. The phenothiazines are by far the most extensively used neuroleptic agents.

1. Phenothiazine Derivatives

Chlorpromazine, the first phenothiazine antipsychotic drug used clinically and still the prototype of this chemical class, is one of the most extensively used drugs in medical practice. During the past ten years, nearly fifty million patients have received chlorpromazine (2). Phenothiazine neuroleptic agents may be subdivided according to the structure of their side chain into aliphatic, piperidine and piperazine derivatives which exhibit certain qualitative and quantitative differences in activity and side effects (see Table 1). For example, the piperidine derivatives have antipsychotic activity equal to chlorpromazine (an aliphatic derivative) but they lack antiemetic activity and cause fewer extrapyramidal side effects than other derivatives. This is of clinical significance in choosing the most effective agent that will exhibit the least number of side effects in a particular patient.

a. Major Pharmacological Effects

Although numerous pharmacological effects are produced by the phenothiazine derivatives, those of major therapeutic significance are their antipsychotic and antiemetic effects.

Antipsychotic activity results from chemical action on subcortical regions of the brainstem which control behavioral and emotional responses. A primary action of blocking the afferent sensory collateral fibers which enter the reticular activating system in the brainstem and a secondary action of depression of various hypothalamic nuclei result in an effective indifference to environmental stimuli, a decrease in spontaneous movement and emotional quieting without a depression of cortical activity. These agents merely decrease the qualitative degree of sensory inputs, particularly those through which activation of the reticular formation may result in aggressive behavior.

Basic, normal behavioral patterns, normal intellectual function and cortical integration are not depressed—major distinguishing characteristics between the neuroleptic agents and the general CNS depressants such as the barbiturates. In contrast to the mental confusion produced in psychotic patients with barbiturate-induced sleep therapy, chlorpromazine significantly reduces mental confusion and agitation. Because of the selective affinity of these agents for those subcortical regions of the brainstem controlling emotional and behavioral responses, the neuroleptic drugs produce a state in which the patient is calm, his thinking is improved, his intellectual and cortical functions are intact and he now becomes responsive to psychotherapy. Although the decrease in sensory inputs reaching the cortex results in a "subdued cortex" and drowsiness, the patient may be aroused easily from this "semi-sedated" state. However, the "subdued cortex" is more sensitive to the depressant effects of agents such as the barbiturates which directly depress the cerebral cortex and reticular activating system. This is most likely the mechanism involved in the potentiated state of CNS depression occurring with combinations of either a barbiturate (or non-barbiturate) sedative-hypnotic agent or a narcotic analgesic and a phenothiazine.

All of the phenothiazine derivatives except the piperidine derivatives are effective antiemetic agents at doses below those required for antipsychotic activity. Since this effect is produced by a direct depression of the chemo-receptor trigger zone in the medulla, the phenothiazines are most useful in the treatment of nausea and vomiting of psychic or organic origin. They are relatively ineffective in the treatment of nausea and vomiting of motion sickness or emesis resulting from local irritation of the gastrointestinal tract.

The actions of the phenothiazine neuroleptic agents on other regions of the brainstem and peripheral autonomic nervous system result in a number of effects which generally are considered to be side effects of these agents.

b. Side Effects and Adverse Reactions

The major side effects produced by the phenothiazine derivatives may be divided into four general categories: 1) effects associated with autonomic blocking action centrally and peripherally, 2) extrapyramidal effects, 3) hypersensitivity reactions, and 4) neuroendocrinologic effects.

One of the more prominent side effects of the phenothiazines is postural hypotension and/or arterial hypotension which results from the central and peripheral adrenolytic actions of these compounds. Centrally, the hypothalamic sympathetic regulatory nuclei and the medullary vasomotor center are depressed; peripherally, the alpha-adrenergic receptors are blocked, particularly by the aliphatic side-chain phenothiazine derivatives. Normal cardiovascular reflex mechanisms such as the carotid sinus vasopressor reflex are depressed significantly. The central depression of the vasomotor center and a peripheral direct depression of vascular smooth muscle result in a phenothiazine-induced vasodilatation. Patients with cardiovascular diseases or impairment, e.g., arteriosclerosis, as frequently seen in the elderly, are particularly susceptible to these effects; likewise, in debilitated patients the hypotensive actions would be greatly enhanced and may result in a hypotensive crisis and other serious complications. The dentist should be aware that patients taking these drugs are particularly susceptible to hypotension and orthostatic cardiovascular collapse, especially at the beginning of phenothiazine therapy or as the degree of physical debilitation increases. Because of the block of alpha-adrenergic receptors, hypotensive crisis in the patient receiving these agents is most difficult to treat. Use of epinephrine would by akathisia and typical parkinsonian-like symptoms. The dystonic syndrome (face, neck, tongue syndrome) occurs more frequently in men and children. This syndrome is of particular interest to the dental practitioner. It is characterized by mandibular tics, protrusion of the tongue, hypertonicity of the muscles of the face and neck with an impairment of speech and swallowing, inability to register centric occlusion, oculogyric spasms, torticollis, tonic twitching and contraction of the trunk muscles. This syndrome may involve the trigeminal nuclei and may be mistaken for a problem of dental origin. The characteristic mandibular tics and spasms of the muscles in the region of the temporomandibular joint and the neck might be mistaken by the physician and the unwary dentist as a problem resulting from one of the many causative factors of temporomandibular joint disorders, a third molar infection or even diagnosed as trigeminal neuralgia. These effects may be more severe and occur more frequently in patients with various debilitating diseases. Most of the extrapyramidal effects are reversible and may be treated with varying degrees of success with centrally acting anticholinergic agents. The use of anticholinergic co-medication would enhance the peripheral anticholinergic actions of the phenothiazines and either may lead to the previously described oral syndrome or increase the severity of an existent xerostomia and associated oral problems.

The most serious side effects produced by the phenothiazines result from hypersensitivity reactions. Intrahepatic obstructive jaundice occurs in more than 4% of the patients taking chlorpromazine, but the frequency varies with other phenothiazine derivatives. Bone marrow depression resulting in an initial stage of leukopenia and subsequent progression to agranulocytosis is a serious hypersensitivity reaction produced by the phenothiazine agents. Patients exhibiting such reactions are predisposed to infections of all types. Concurrent treatment with agents which reduce white blood cells or co-existent disease and severe debilitation increase the susceptibility to phenothiazine-induced leukopenia. Agranulocytosis may be fatal with a greater than 40% mortality rate. Other hypersensitivity reactions are exhibited as various dermatological reactions such as photosensitivity of the skin, alterations in skin pigmentation, and a host of other characteristic skin reactions. Many of these reactions also may be evident in the oral cavity (stomatitis medicamentosa).

The effects produced by chlorpromazine and other phenothiazines on endocrine responses are produced through depression of the hypothalamic-hypophysial system and include the following: suppression of the release of pituitary gonadotropins, somatotrophic hormone, ACTH, be contraindicated, since its vasoconstrictive effects would be blocked while its beta-adrenergic effects (vasodepressor effects) would be enhanced; epinephrine would cause a further decrease in blood pressure—i.e., epinephrine reversal. Although the problem is less serious, several reports have indicated that the *local* vasoconstrictive effects of epinephrine also may be antagonized by chlorpromazine.

The phenothiazines exhibit peripheral anticholinergic actions similar to those produced by atropine-like compounds. This action results in the side effects of increase in pulse rate, tachycardia, constipation and difficulty in micturition, stuffy nose, blurred vision, a peculiar gray pallor of the skin, and xerostomia. Phenothiazine-induced xerostomia is produced by the atropine-like action of blocking the peripheral cholinergic receptors and is not the result of any pathological changes in the salivary glands. This action is quite prominent and has been described as part of the "oral syndrome" frequently produced by these agents. The oral syndrome is described as dry mouth, diffuse redness of the oral mucosa, the various lesions of stomatitis medicamentosa, denture stomatitis, white or black hairy tongue or bald beefy red tongue, formation of a thick white pseudomembrane, loosened dentures frequently associated with vesicular lesions in the mouth or on the tongue, and an increased susceptibility to candida and other oral infections. This condition is increased in severity by anticholinergic agents which are employed frequently in treating the extrapyramidal side effects produced by the phenothiazine tranquilizers. If the patient's medication cannot be changed to another neuroleptic agent with less anticholinergic activity, hourly mouth rinses or lemon-glycerine swabs may provide some degree of comfort. Unless contraindicated, potassium chloride (300 mg orally three times daily) may be effective in increasing the quantity of saliva. The use of cholinergic stimulants to counteract the dry mouth generally would be contraindicated in these debilitated patients.

The general effects of the phenothiazine derivatives on the basal ganglia and associated nuclei result in the extrapyramidal side effects produced by these agents. These effects may occur with relatively high frequency, being as high as 10% in the case of the phenothiazine derivatives. These effects are particularly frequent with high doses of the phenothiazines and are particularly predominant with those derivatives containing a piperazine side chain. The susceptibility to these effects varies with the age and sex of the patient. In elderly patients of both sexes and women of all ages the extrapyramidal effects are generally characterized and antidiuretic hormone. It should be noted that the patient's ability to respond to stressful stimuli is severely impaired. A depressant effect on the hypothalamic thermoregulatory center results in the poikilothermic effects produced by the phenothiazine derivatives. Body temperature tends to take on that of the environment. The debilitated patient taking these agents may die from severe hypothermia or hyperthermia unless the environmental temperature is controlled.

c. Drug Interactions and Contraindications

Phenothiazine derivatives interact with a number of other drugs having effects on the central nervous system. The CNS depressant effects of the barbiturates, non-barbiturate sedative-hypnotic drugs, narcotic analgesics, and alcohol are potentiated.

Although low doses of the phenothiazines do not depress respiration, increasingly larger doses progressively may depress respiration. The respiratory depressant action of other agents such as the barbiturates and narcotic analgesics is potentiated by the phenothiazine derivatives. Both the systemic activity and toxicity of local anesthetics are potentiated by the phenothiazines. A very serious drug interaction resulting in hypotensive crisis and severe extrapyramidal side effects occurs when a monamine oxidase inhibitor-type antidepressant is given concurrently or shortly after cessation of phenothiazine therapy.

A significant potentiation of the CNS depressant effects of alcohol by the phenothiazines may result from the inhibition of alcohol dehydrogenase by these tranquilizers. Therefore, the combination of a phenothiazine with any other CNS depressant requires that the dose of each be reduced from 1/2 to 2/3 of the usual single dose. Whether or not the phenothiazine agents enhance the analgesia produced by narcotic analgesic drugs is controversial; it has been reported that the combination of promethazine with meperidine actually results in a reduction of the analgesic activity, i.e., an anti-analgesic effect (3). However, potentiation of the toxicities and side effects (respiratory depression, hypotension, etc.) of both groups of drugs is indisputable.

The hypotensive effects of agents which lower blood pressure (e.g., antihypertensive drugs such as reserpine, adrenolytic agents, diuretics, and so on) are potentiated by the phenothiazines. Therefore, the phenothiazine derivatives are contraindicated in patients taking antihypertensive drugs or who have a labile blood pressure.

Whereas these are the usual interactions occurring in patients relatively free of major somatic diseases, the practitioner must recognize that all of these problems may be intensified greatly and that additional interactions may occur in patients with impaired homeostatic mechanisms.

2. Other Neuroleptic Tranquilizers

Following the discovery of the beneficial effect of the phenothiazine neuroleptic agents, the continuing search for new agents with enhanced antipsychotic activity and diminished side effects resulted in two additional chemical classes of antipsychotic drugs which are presently used clinically, the butyrophenone and thioxanthene derivatives. Both classes are effective antipsychotic agents and are used as alternatives to the phenothiazines. These agents exhibit certain advantages over the phenothiazine neuroleptic agents in certain clinical situations and are used mainly in cases refractory to the phenothiazines or in patients who cannot tolerate certain adverse effects of the phenothiazines. In general, the major pharmacological effects, side effects, toxicities, mechanisms of action and therapeutic uses are similar to those for the phenothiazines; however, certain differences are exhibited which are of interest.

The thioxanthene derivatives exhibit effects most similar to those of the phenothiazine neuroleptic agents. Although the side effects may be slightly less frequent and severe with these derivatives, their overall adverse effects quite closely parallel those produced by the phenothiazine antipsychotic drugs. As with the phenothiazines, adverse effects include extrapyramidal effects, lowering convulsive seizure threshold, peripheral anticholinergic effects (nasal congestion, tachycardia, xerostomia and other oral problems, and so on), central and peripheral adrenolytic effects, alterations in endocrine hormone secretion and other side effects described for the phenothiazine agents. The same contraindications, cautions and drug interactions previously discussed for the phenothiazines also apply for the thioxanthene derivatives. Thus, the dentist should consider the patient treated with these derivatives in the same way as he would those treated with the phenothiazines.

The pharmacological effects of the butyrophenone derivatives may be summarized briefly by comparing their activity with the phenothiazine neuroleptic agents. In general, these compounds produce similar effects with the following exceptions: (a) they are considerably more potent; (b) they do not exhibit any peripheral anticholinergic effects; (c) they do not cause any alterations in endocrine hormone secretion; (d) they interfere with central adrenergic mechanisms but exhibit little peripheral adrenolytic effects and are less likely to cause arterial hypotension and orthostatic hypotension. This latter aspect makes these compounds useful alternatives to the phenothiazines in elderly patients and patients with cardiovascular abnormalities. Other effects, both those of therapeutic benefit as well as adverse effects, are practically identical with those of the phenothiazines. The extrapyramidal side effects produced by these agents occur with great frequency and severity (see Table 1). Xerostomia and the oral syndrome associated with the phenothiazine derivatives generally would not be a problem in patients taking these agents, but the dystonic syndrome and related extrapyramidal effects may comprise serious problems for both the dentist and the physician. If antiparkinson drugs (i.e., centrally acting anticholinergic agents) are used in treating the extrapyramidal side effects, xerostomia and associated oral problems should be expected.

B. Anxiolytic Sedatives

These agents are useful in the treatment of various psychoneurotic states, anxiety states, tension and agitation. This category of drugs (also known as minor tranquilizers) includes the carbamate derivatives, the benzodiazepine derivatives, the diphenylmethane derivatives, and the phenothiazine antihistaminic derivatives (non-neuroleptic agents), e.g., promethazine (Phenergan®). The effects of many of these agents, particularly of the diphenylmethane series, are much more similar to the effects produced by barbiturates than they are to those produced by either the neuroleptic agents or the other groups of anxiolytic sedatives. Although some effects of promethazine are similar to those of the antipsychotic phenothiazine derivatives, the action of promethazine on the central nervous system is quite similar to that of an anxiolytic sedative agent.

The effects produced by the anxiolytic sedatives or "minor tranquilizers" differ from those produced by the neuroleptic "major tranquilizers" in several important respects. A comparison of the pharmacological effects of the anxiolytic sedatives with those of the neuroleptic agents is provided in Table 2. The major pharmacological effects of both the carbamate and benzodiazepine derivatives are summarized and compared in Table 3.

1. Carbamate Derivatives

The carbamate derivatives are the prototype group of anxiolytic sedatives. At present the carbamate derivatives used clinically include meprobamate, carisoprodol, tybamate, mebutamate and chlorphenesin carbamate. Because of the similarity between the pharmacological effects of the carbamate derivatives and those produced by the benzodiazepine derivatives, the major pharmacological activity will be discussed for the prototype carbamate compound, meprobamate. Unless otherwise stated, it may be assumed that the benzodiazepine derivatives have similar pharmacological effects.

a. Pharmacological Effects of Meprobamate

It is generally believed that at usual therapeutic doses meprobamate exerts its action on subcortical areas in the brainstem, in contrast to the action of the barbiturates which in sedative doses act at cortical levels as well as certain levels in the reticular formation. Available information indicates that the primary site of action of meprobamate is in the thalamus and the secondary site of action of this compound is in the limbic system. At higher doses meprobamate also can produce cortical depression with the production of sleep, but there is a large margin between the small doses producing mild sedation and those causing direct cortical depression and sleep. Meprobamate exerts an anti-anxiety action in man at doses below those causing significant direct cortical depression.

Two distinguishing characteristics of the "minor tranquilizer" agents in general, and meprobamate in particular, are their anticonvulsant action and depressant effect on spinal reflex activity. Meprobamate exerts an anticonvulsant activity similar to that produced by trimethadione. It may be an effective adjuvant in the treatment of petit mal epilepsy. It is contraindicated in the treatment of grand mal epilepsy since it aggravates grand mal seizures. Meprobamate acts as a skeletal muscle relaxant by depression of polysynaptic pathways in the spinal cord without affecting monosynaptic pathways. These drugs do not affect the neuromuscular junction and are classified as centrally acting skeletal muscle relaxants. Skeletal muscle relaxant activity is enhanced in some of the carbamate derivatives, e.g., carisoprodol (Soma®). These derivatives produce a sufficient degree of skeletal muscle relaxation, at doses which usually do not cause significant sedation, to be clinically useful in the treatment of some acute musculoskeletal disorders. Meprobamate and other carbamate derivatives also selectively depress internuncial neurones in the brainstem at the thalamic level. It has been postulated that depression of the long internuncial neuronal circuits (reverberating circuits) between the thalamus and the cerebral cortex is the mechanism involved in the anxiolytic action of these compounds (Berger, 1954).

Physical and psychological dependence develop with chronic use of meprobamate, particularly in doses of above 2.4 gms per day (total dose). In an individual physically dependent on meprobamate, withdrawal of the drug produces a syndrome similar to that produced by barbiturate withdrawal (characterized by grand mal seizures). However, the abstinence syndrome is of shorter duration than that which occurs with barbiturates.

b. Therapeutic Uses

The therapeutic usefulness of meprobamate is in the treatment of mild to moderately severe psychoneuroses, anxiety and tension states. Meprobamate and particularly some of the other carbamate derivatives are used frequently as centrally acting skeletal muscle relaxants in the treatment of muscular spasms. These agents may be effective in relieving the skeletal muscle tension and spasms resulting from bruxism or temporomandibular joint dysfunction.

The carbamate derivatives also have been used successfully in the treatment of behavioral disorders in children and in the treatment of chronic alcoholism (5). Meprobamate has been used effectively as a premedication agent for the apprehensive dental patient. Small doses of meprobamate have been used effectively in prosthetic patients with nervous or hyperemotional dispositions during the period of adjustment to the new appliance. Meprobamate and similar minor tranquilizers may be especially useful in the pre-operative sedation of children and elderly individuals who exhibit paradoxical CNS excitatory effects with the barbiturates or in a patient who is allergic to the barbiturates. In addition, the anxiolytic sedatives may be useful in patients who respond to the average dose of other sedative agents such as the barbiturates with excessive drowsiness, sedation, ataxia and "hangover."

c. Major Side Effects and Precautions

Drowsiness, sometimes associated with lethargy and ataxia, is the most prominent side effect produced by meprobamate and similar "minor tranquilizers" and the usual general precautions regarding the use of barbiturate sedative-hypnotic agents are applicable also with the use of the anxiolytic sedatives. In one study, 400 mg of meprobamate impaired driving performance, but the impairment was much less than that caused by 100 mg of secobarbital. When meprobamate is used as a premedicating agent, the dentist should caution the patient about driving an automobile or other vehicles and the operation of dangerous machinery. It is of interest that elderly patients are particularly sensitive to the CNS depressant effects of meprobamate; and occasionally in some patients, especially debilitated patients or patients with cardiovascular disorders, arterial hypotension and susceptibility to orthostatic hypotensive episodes may occur.

The carbamate derivatives can produce allergic reactions occurring in from 0.2 to 3.4% of the patients; these hypersensitivity reactions occur more frequently in patients with a history of allergic conditions. Allergic reactions concerning the oral mucosa (stomatitis medicamentosa) can be produced by meprobamate and occur most frequently (6). Even anaphylaxis and anaphylactoid-type reactions have been reported following the administration of meprobamate (7). Other allergic manifestations include urticaria, various skin rashes, peripheral edema and ecchymoses, angioneurotic edema, fever, bronchial spasms, hypotensive crises, anuria and proctitis. Additional side effects produced by meprobamate include dizziness, headache, gastrointestinal discomfort and disturbances, chills, fever, paresthesia, glossitis and dry mouth.

The overall toxicity of the anxiolytic sedatives is much less than that of the neuroleptic tranquilizers or of the barbiturates.

d. Drug Interactions

Meprobamate and other minor tranquilizers enhance the CNS depressant effects of a number of agents such as alcohol, barbiturate and non-barbiturate sedative-hypnotic agents, phenothiazine derivatives, and any other group of CNS depressants. With alcohol there is a potentiation, or at least more than an additive effect, of CNS depression resulting in marked drowsiness or hypnosis. Meprobamate has been shown to increase the impairment of motor ability produced by alcohol (8). There is also of the pharmacology of these compounds.

b. Therapeutic Uses

The therapeutic effectiveness and indications for the use of benzodiazepine derivatives are similar to those for meprobamate. As a premedication agent either diazepam or chlordiazepoxide has a slow onset of action (8 hours) when given orally. Therefore, the use of this agent to allay apprehension prior to a dental procedure would require that the agent be given the day prior to the appointment as well as on the day of the appointment. When these agents are given by intramuscular injection, their onset of action is relatively fast (approximately 30-45 minutes). The use of diazepam as an anxiolytic sedative during dental procedures is growing in popularity. The interested reader can consult the following reference for a detailed discussion of the use of diazepam during both oral surgical and routine dental procedures (13).

c. Side Effects and Adverse Reactions

The benzodiazepine derivatives produce all of the side effects exhibited by the carbamate derivatives plus several additional side effects. In general, the benzodiazepines exhibit a greater overall toxicity than do the carbamate derivatives.

One of the major differences between the effects produced by the benzodiazepine derivatives and the meprobamate-like anxiolytic sedatives is the action of the former on the peripheral autonomic nervous system. Benzodiazepines exhibit weak to moderate anticholinergic activity peripherally. For this reason these compounds are contraindicated in patients who have narrow angle glaucoma. Xerostomia and associated oral problems should be expected.

In general, doses of the benzodiazepine derivatives which produce anxiolytic effects without marked CNS depression do not impair performance significantly. However, at higher doses these compounds may affect reflexes and cause side effects of lethargy and drowsiness. From a number of studies it is debatable whether the benzodiazepine derivatives impair driving performance to a greater extent, to a lesser extent or to the same extent as meprobamate and similar carbamate derivatives.

The benzodiazepine derivatives produce some undesirable effects in elderly patients. These individuals apparently are very susceptible to the

CNS depressant effects of this group of compounds and even at low therapeutic doses hypotension may occur frequently. These patients are predisposed to attacks of syncope and orthostatic hypotension. Another effect resulting from benzodiazepine compounds, particularly in elderly patients, is a paradoxical CNS excitatory reaction similar to that occurring with the barbiturate sedative-hypnotic agents. This effect is accompanied by confusion, inebriation, delirium and ataxia. This reaction has been reported mainly in elderly patients taking chlordiazepoxide.

d. Drug Interactions and Precautions

A number of drug interaction problems occur with these compounds. Combination of a benzodiazepine derivative with one of the other CNS depressant agents causes at least additive depressant effects and generally potentiation of the CNS depressant actions of both drugs occurs.

Adverse behavioral reactions as well as excessive CNS depression have occurred when the benzodiazepine derivatives are given to patients concurrently taking barbiturates, phenothiazine neuroleptic agents or certain antidepressant drugs. These three groups of psychoactive drugs are used extensively and also may be indicated and used by the dying patient as well as by the "somatically healthy" dental patient. The dental practitioner must be well aware of such drug interactions so that a benzodiazepine derivative is not given to a patient concurrently taking one or more of these other psychoactive drugs.

C. Antidepressant Agents

This subclass of psychopharmacological agents consists of two major groups of compounds, the monoamine oxidase inhibitor (MAOI) antidepressants and the tricyclic antidepressants, used clinically for their therapeutic effectiveness in the treatment of various pathological depressed states. The MAOI antidepressants were the first compounds used specifically in the treatment of mental depression. These agents produce profound alterations in catecholamine metabolism and storage of biogenic amines in both the central and peripheral nervous systems. The MAOI antidepressant drugs produce numerous untoward reactions; serious drug interactions occur with almost every drug class and fatal interactions have occurred frequently with combinations of the MAOI antidepressants and several classes of drugs. The availability of the less toxic and clinically more effective tricyclic antidepressants fortunately has resulted in a decrease in the clinical use of the MAOI antidepressants.

The tricyclic antidepressants are the most extensively used agents clinically and generally the MAOI's are reserved for the treatment of depressive states which are refractory to treatment with the tricyclic antidepressants. Both groups of antidepressants are used clinically in the treatment of a variety of depressed states including reactive (situational) depression, endogenous depressed states including manic-depressive psychoses, organic conditions such as senile depression, phobic-anxiety states, neurotic depressions and other types of psychiatric disorders. They are most effective in mild to severe endogenous or retarded depressions.

The discovery of the effectiveness of chlorpromazine in certain psychiatric disorders provided the basis for a number of theories regarding the biochemical etiology of mental diseases. In the same manner a number of hypotheses have been formulated which state that mental depression may be related to a decrease in brain monoamines such as norepinephrine, serotonin, and dopamine, particularly at their respective receptors in the brain. The evidence supporting these hypotheses is inconclusive at present. However, both the MAOI and tricyclic antidepressants increase the amount of free norepinephrine at the adrenergic receptors in the CNS; this action may be related to their CNS stimulating effects and antidepressant activity. Some of the pharmacological effects (and related side effects) produced by the MAOI antidepressants are significantly different from those occurring with the tricyclic antidepressants, as shown in Table 4.

Whether or not these agents should be used by the dying patient is dependent upon a number of factors, such as the attending physician's judgment and experience with the clinical use of these drugs, the type of terminal illness and so on. Since these compounds have been used in the treatment of senile depression and certain reactive depressions, use most likely would be indicated in the treatment of severe depression in the terminal patient who is expected to live for several months or longer. Certain chemical subgroups of the MAOI antidepressant drugs have been used for a number of other pathological conditions besides mental diseases. Some derivatives have been used as analgesics in patients with progressive neoplastic disease or for their anticoagulant activity in depressed patients suffering from coronary thrombosis or peripheral clotting disorders (14).

Although the justification for the use of these agents in conditions in which less toxic and equally effective drugs might be employed may be severely questioned, the preceding examples indicate that these agents may be used in various pathological states in which their use usually would not be indicated or expected. Therefore, it is not unlikely that these agents may be prescribed for the dying patient, although there is no conceivable rationale for the use of these drugs in the treatment of oral disease. The numerous side effects and serious, sometimes fatal, drug interaction problems occurring with both groups of antidepressants increase both the risks and difficulties encountered in the treatment of oral disease in patients taking these drugs. As described previously for the neuroleptic tranquilizers and the anxiolytic sedatives, many of the side effects exhibited by the antidepressant drugs may be manifested in the oro-facial region of the body or may be the primary etiological factor in the patient's oral problem(s). Severe drug interactions occur between the antidepressant drugs and those compounds which normally would be used by the dentist in treating the patient's oral diseases. Therefore, these compounds will be discussed from the standpoint of their major side effects and drug interaction problems relevant to the patient's oral care. The reader is referred to numerous articles in the pharmacological literature for an extensive discussion of the pharmacological effects and clinical use of these agents in various types of mental depression.

1. Monoamine Oxidase Inhibitor-Type Antidepressant Drugs

The agents presently used clinically are tranylcypromine (Parnate®), isocarboxazid (Marplan®), nialamid (Niamid®), phenelzine (Nardil®), and pagyline (Eutonyl®). These agents are used for their antidepressant effects with the exception of pargyline which is used clinically as an antihypertensive agent.

a. Pharmacological Effects, Side Effects and Adverse Reactions

These compounds are effective inhibitors of not only monoamine oxidase but also a number of other oxidative enzymes including the hepatic drug metabolizing enzymes. Inhibition of monoamine oxidase, which is involved with the intraneuronal metabolism of biogenic amines, results in the accumulation of serotonin, norepinephrine, dopamine epinephrine and various precursors of these amines within the brain, peripheral adrenergic nerve endings and liver. Although these effects are probably related to the antidepressant action of these compounds, it has not been established unequivocally that inhibition of MAOI is the mechanism by which the antidepressant effects are produced. However, there is little doubt that a number of the side effects and drug interaction problems associated with these compounds are the result of inhibition of monoamine oxidase and other enzymes. Inhibition of the hepatic drug metabolizing enzymes is the basis for several of the drug interaction problems occurring with the MAOI antidepressant agents.

The major side effects produced by the MAOI antidepressant drugs are adverse CNS excitatory reactions and alterations in autonomic function manifested mainly as effects on the cardiovascular system. The most prominent action of these compounds on the cardiovascular system is the production of hypotension. Patients taking any of the MAOI antidepressants are predisposed to arterial hypotension, particularly orthostatic hypotension. Several hypotheses have been offered regarding the mechanism(s) involved in these cardiovascular effects. The theories have included ganglionic blocking activity and, as indicated by more recent evidence, a block of the nerve impulse-induced release of norepinephrine from the adrenergic nerve endings. These drugs affect the intragranular pool of norepinephrine which is released by the nerve action potential but apparently do not affect the release of norepinephrine from the "drug-releasable" cytoplasmic pool. Cardiovascular reflexes such as the carotid sinus vasopressor (baroreceptor) reflex are impaired.

The effects resemble those of peripheral adrenergic blockade. Predisposition to postural hypotension and the lack of compensatory cardiovascular reflexes may result in hypotensive crises, particularly in the debilitated patient; the dentist should be aware of this problem and exercise the usual precautions, particularly in the ambulatory patient. Additional side effects are related to the peripheral autonomic actions of these compounds and include dryness of the oral mucosa, hyperhidrosis, hot flashes, difficulty in micturition, diarrhea, constipation, blurred vision and impotence. Dry mouth is a frequently occurring side effect of the MAOI antidepressants; since depressed states alone are frequently associated with a dry mouth syndrome, the use of one of these agents would increase the severity of the existing xerostomia and may result in more severe oral complications. Excessive CNS stimulation, hepatotoxic reactions, blood dyscrasias and allergic reactions have occurred as side effects of these drugs.

b. Drug Interaction Problems

The MAOI antidepressant drugs are associated with more severe and frequent drug interactions than any of the other psychopharmacological agents used clinically. The types of drugs which cause adverse effects when administered concurrently with a MAOI antidepressant are varied and numerous; intolerance to any other drug acting on the central nervous some indication that the use of an anxiolytic sedative agent concurrently with an antidepressant drug, particularly a monoamine oxidase inhibitor, increases the incidence of adverse reactions.

2. Benzodiazepine Derivatives

The benzodiazepine derivatives are the newest members of the anxiolytic sedatives. The first member and prototype compound of this series, chlordiazepoxide (Librium®), has been administered to more patients during the past 6 years than any other single compound (9). There are two additional benzodiazepine derivatives, diazepan (Valium®) and oxazepan (Serax®), *both of which currently* are used for their anxiolytic properties.

The capacity of the benzodiazepine derivatives to exert anxiolytic activity at doses which do not affect alertness indicates that these agents act on subcortical structures of the brainstem. The marked sensitivity of the limbic lobe structures to the benzodiazepines as well as the anxiolytic action of these agents at doses which do not alter consciousness or alertness indicates that the limbic system is their primary site of action; the benzodiazepines exert a depressant effect on the limbic lobe structures at doses which do not depress the cerebral cortex or brainstem reticular formation. Their secondary site of action would appear to be the hypothalamus and/or thalamus, both of which are depressed by the benzodiazepine derivates.

a. Pharmacological Effects

In general, chlordiazepoxide and other benzodiazepine anxiolytic sedatives produce pharmacological effects differing only in minor quantitative aspects from the effects produced by meprobamate (see Table 3). Their pharmacological properties best exemplify the effects produced by "true" anxiolytic sedative agents ("minor tranquilizers"). Prominent anxiolytic effects may be achieved at therapeutic doses of chlordiazepoxide or diazepam which do not affect alertness or produce hypnosis, oversedation or ataxia (10, 11). In this respect they are more similar to the phenothiazine "major tranquilizers" than to the carbamate derivatives which more closely resemble the barbiturates in pharmacological properties. The anticonvulsant activity and skeletal muscle relaxant properties of the benzodiazepine derivatives are more pronounced than those of meprobamate. The reader is referred to the review article by Zbinden and Randall (12) for a more extensive discussion system is to be expected in the patient taking these antidepressant agents. A *partial* listing of some of the more severe drug interactions frequently occurring with the MAOI's is given in Table 5. Particular attention should be given to the serious and possibly fatal interactions occurring when any narcotic analgesic, but especially meperidine, is given to patients taking a MAOI antidepressant drug; likewise, fatal interactions, have occurred with other CNS depressant drugs (see Table 5). The only way to avoid drug interactions with any degree of certainty in patients receiving these antidepressant drugs is *to avoid using any other drug.* The only possible exception to this is the use of local anesthetics, with or without vasoconstrictors; great care must be exercised in aspirating to avoid systemic injection of the local anesthetic since the systemic toxicity of these drugs is increased markedly by the MAOI antidepressants. The central effects, but usually not the peripheral effects, of the directly-acting sympathomimetic amines such as epinephrine and norepinephrine also are potentiated by this group of antidepressant drugs. Very serious and fatal drug interactions resulting in hypertensive crisis, intracranial bleeding and death have occurred with indirectly-acting sympathomimetic amines such as amphetamine and tyramine in patients taking one of the MAOI's. A number of deaths have resulted from ingestion of certain foods (cheeses, wines, broad beans) which contain tyramine or dopamine by patients taking tranycypromine.

2. Tricyclic Antidepressant Drugs

The widely used agents belonging to this group of drugs are the dibenzazepine derivates, imipramine (Tofranil®) and desmethylimipramine (Pertofran®, Norpramin®) and the dibenzocycloheptadiene derivatives, amitriptyline (Elavil®). These compounds are similar, both structurally and pharmacologically, to the phenothiazine neuroleptic drugs. In reality they may be classified as "stimulating tranquilizers." They exert a tranquilizing effect in the "normal" patient similar to that produced by the phenothiazine tranquilizers; but in the patient with mental depression, their CNS stimulating (antidepressant) effects are apparent and useful clinically in treating these patients. Because of this dual-type action, the clinician might classify these agents as "tranquilizer-antidepressant" drugs. Indeed, most of the effects, side effects, and drug interactions discussed for the phenothiazine neuroleptic agents can be applied without modification to the tricyclic antidepressant agents. The major differences between the tricyclic antidepressants and the phenothiazine tranquilizers are mainly quantitative.

The major side effects produced by the tricyclic antidepressant rugs are essentially the same as those described for the phenothiazine derivatives. These agents exhibit peripheral anticholinergic activity (atropine-like action) which is quantitatively more prominent than that occurring with the phenothiazines. Dry mouth, tachycardia, blurred vision and other effects resulting from the atropine-like action of these drugs occur frequently. Therefore, the dentist should expect that patients taking these drugs would have xerostomia and related oral problems. As with the phenothiazines, postural hypotension, especially in the elderly or in debilitated patients, occurs frequently as a side effect of the tricyclic antidepressants and requires that the usual precautions be taken in treating these patients. Parkinson-like symptoms and other extrapyramidal effects similar to those produced by the phenothiazines also occur with the tricyclic antidepressants; but these effects usually occur less frequently and are less severe with these agents than with the phenothiazines.

Major drug interaction problems occurring with the tricyclic antidepressants are similar to those for the phenothiazine tranquilizers. The anticholinergic effects of atropine-like drugs are increased by the concurrent use of a tricyclic antidepressant drug. The tricyclic antidepressants block the uptake of monoamines into the nerve ending resulting in potentiation of both the central and peripheral effects of injected norepinephrine and epinephrine. The use of these catecholamines topically as hemostatic or gingival retraction agents is contraindicated. The effects of both CNS depressants and CNS stimulants (e.g., amphetamine) are potentiated by the tricyclic antidepressants. Significant potentiation of the respiratory depression produced by the barbiturates and narcotic analgesics occurs and would be a serious drug interaction problem in the patient with existing respiratory disorders. Serious toxic effects resembling atropine toxicity occur when tricyclic antidepressants are given concurrently, or within several weeks following discontinuation of therapy, with the MAOI antidepressant agents. Some of these reactions have been fatal.

II. Narcotic Analgesics

The narcotic analgesics include the crude drug, opium, all the many galenical preparations of opium, as well as opium's alkaloids and the many more semi-synthetic and fully synthetic derivatives and substitutes of morphine (the standard strong analgesic and the prototype of this drug class). Morphine administered in the appropriate dosage can relieve any kind of pain without causing the patient to lose consciousness.

Pharmacological Effects

The best known and desirable effects of morphine are those which result from the drug's action at various sites in the central nervous system. Morphine is known to reduce pain in at least three ways: 1) it raises the so-called "pain perception threshold"; 2) it reduces the reaction to pain; and 3) it promotes sedation and sleep (which, in itself, facilitates both one and two). All evidence would indicate that the major factor is the drug's ability to reduce the emotional reaction to pain, i.e., the anxiety induced by the anticipation of pain. The morphine-treated patient is not physiologically free of pain, but he is inattentive or unaware of the pain. He could not care less about the pain in the drug-induced false state of well-being known as euphoria. The site of morphine's analgesic action may be the complex reciprocal pathways between the thalamic and frontal cortex levels of the CNS.

Morphine produces an array of side effects as a result of simultaneous stimulation and depression of the entire central axis. Some of the more important effects clinically are: miosis, emesis, respiratory depression, "cough center" depression, anti-diuresis, inhibition of ACTH secretion, and monosynaptic reflex enhancement accompanied by polysynaptic reflex depression.

Morphine leads to an insignificant incidence of cardiovascular effects in the patient who is not debilitated and who is free of CNS depressants. The dying patient, however, may be expected to manifest exaggerated depression of the cardiovascular system due to morphine's depressant action upon the vasomotor center and also the peripheral vascular smooth muscle (partly due to histamine release).

Morphine's other predictable, distressing untoward effects, which appear while the drug is relieving the dying patient's pain and suffering, are: urinary retention, constipation, spasm of the sphincter of Oddi, and, most importantly and unfortunately the development of tolerance to the desirable effects of the drug. With progressively increasing dosages in order to surmount the tolerance, physical dependence upon the drug is the inevitable result. This is perhaps the most challenging and awesome task of the attending clinician, i. e., to juggle with exact precision the complex, individually manifested and incalculable factors of the patient's terminating condition, degree of severe pain, the rate of tolerance development to the analgesic action of the drug, the appearance of drug toxicities, and so on.

Contraindications and Dangerous Interactions

It should not be surprising that a patient with emphysema, who is having a difficult time maintaining an adequate respiratory exchange in the non-drugged state, does not require more than minute amounts of a narcotic analgesic before respiratory failure occurs. In addition, morphine contracts the bronchiolar smooth muscle, increases the flow of respiratory tract fluid and depresses the cough reflex, an ominous combination in the dying patient.

The administration of morphine to the dying patient with a history of bronchial asthma could cause the patient's premature death.

The rate of morphine biotransformation in man is determined mainly by the relative amount of functional hepatic tissue present. Hence, in a dying patient with hepatic disease, the dosage must be reduced accordingly or the drug may be contraindicated.

The patient with hypothyroid disease, in addition to his terminal disorder, must be given narcotic analgesics only with *extreme caution*, because the combination of depressed cellular functions will augment the depressant effects of the drug.

The narcotic analgesics are known to interact unfavorably with a number of other drugs, especially those which a dying patient conceivably may be taking, such as: 1) the monoamine-oxidase inhibitor-type of antidepressant agent; 2) the barbiturate or non-barbiturate sedative hypnotics; or 3) the neuroleptic drugs and the anxiolytic sedatives.

The rapidly lethal interaction which occurs within minutes after administering meperidine (Demerol) to a patient taking tranylcypromine (Parnate) is well documented in the literature. The other CNS depressants mentioned interact with the narcotic analgesics to enhance the drug-induced depression. Such results are, by far, more apt to occur in the debilitated dying patient.

Let it be understood, nonetheless, that many of these known contraindications to the use of narcotic analgesics may be rationally set aside by the clinician when it becomes his major concern . . . "to provide relief, not restoration to useful life (15)."

References

1. J. F. Delay, P. Deniker, and J. M. Harl, "Utilization en Therapeutique Psychiatrique d'une Phenothiazine d'Action Centrale Elective (4560 R. P.)," *Annales MedicoPsychologiques, 110:*112-117, 1952.
2. T. A. Ban, *Psychopharmacology*, Baltimore: Williams and Wilkins, Co., 1969.
3. J. Moore and J. W. Dundee, "Alterations in Response to Somatic Pain Associated with Anaesthesia: V. The Effect of Promethazine," *British Journal of Anaesthesia, 33:*3-8, 1961.
4. F. M. Berger, "The Pharmacological Properties of 2-Methyl-2-N-Propyl-1,3 Propanediol Dicarbamate (Miltown) a New Interneuronal Blocking Agent," *Journal of Pharmacology and Experimental Therapeutics, 112:*412, 1954.
5. F. M. Berger and B. J. Ludwig, "Meprobamate and Related Compounds," *Psychopharmacological Agents*, edited by M. Gordon, New York: Academic Press, 1964.
6. *Accepted Dental Therapeutics*, 33rd Edition, Chicago: American Dental Association, 1970.
7. E. V. Adline et al., "Fatal Reaction Following Ingestion of Meprobamate," *Archives of Internal Medicine*, Chicago, 102:484, 1958.
8. G. A. Zirkle, O. B. McAtee, P. O. King, and R. Van Dyke, "Meprobamate and Small Amounts of Alcohol: Effects on Human Ability, Coordination and Judgment," *Journal of the American Medical Association, 173:*1823, 1960.
9. T. A. Ban, *Op. Cit.*
10. S. E. Svenson and R. Hamilton, "A Critique of Overemphasis on Side Effects with the Psychotropic Drugs: An Analysis of 18,000 Chlordiazepoxide-Treated Cases," *Current Therapeutic Research, 8:*455, 1966.
11. J. M. Tobin, I. F. Bird, and D. E. Boyle, "Preliminary Evaluation of Librium (R05-0690) in the Treatment of Anxiety Reactions," *Diseases of the Nervous System, 21:*11, 1960.
12. G. Zbinden and L. Randall, "Pharmacology of Benzodiazepines: Laboratory and Clinical Correlations," *Advances in Pharmacology, 5:*213-291, 1967.
13. E. S. Baird and G. D. Flowerdew, "Intravenous Diazepam in Conservative Dentistry," *British Dental Journal, 128:*11, 1970.
14. T. A. Ban, *Op. Cit.*
15. *Drugs of Choice, 1970-1971*, edited by W. Modell, St. Louis: C. V. Mosby, 1970, p. 216.

Additional References

1. P. B. Bradley, "Phenothiazine Derivatives," *Physiological Pharmacology*, Vol. 1, Part A. edited by W. S. Roos and F. G. Hofman, New York: Academic Press, 1963, p. 417.
2. F. Th. v. Brucke, O. Hornkiewicz, and E. G. Sigg, *The Pharmacology of Psychotherapeutic Drugs*, New York: Spring-Verlag, 1969.
3. L. S. Goodman and A. Gilman, *The Pharmacological Basis of Therapeutics*, 4th Edition, New York: The Macmillan Co., 1970.
4. A. Grollman and E. F. Grollman, *Pharmacology and Therapeutics*, 7th Edition, Philadelphia: Lea and Febiger, 1970.
5. P. A. J. Janssen, "The Pharmacology of Haloperiodol," *International Journal of Neuropsychiatry*, 3:(S1), S10-S18, 1967.
6. E. Leer, *Chemistry and Applied Pharmacology of Tranquilizers*, Springfield: Charles C. Thomas, 1966.
7. P. V. Petersen and M. I. Nielsen, "Thioxanthene Derivatives," *Psychopharmacological Agents*, edited by M. Gordon, New York: Academic Press, 1964.
9. V. P. Whittaker cit. D. Richter, "Biochemical Mechanisms Related to the Site of Action of Psychotropic Drugs," *Neuropsychopharmacology*, Vol. II, edited by E. Rothlin, Amsterdam: Elservier Publishing Co., 1961, p. 422.
10. V. C. Sutherland, *A Synopsis of Pharmacology*, 2nd Edition, Philadelphia: W. B. Saunders Co., 1970.

TABLE 1
Major Adverse Effects of Neuroleptic Agents (Antipsychotic Drugs)

Drug Class	Frequent	Occasional	Rare
A. PHENOTHIAZINES			
1. Aliphatic derivatives Chlorpromazine (THORAZINE) Promazine (SPARINE) Triflupromazine (VESPRIN)	Oversedation; postural hypotension; anticholinergic effects	Cholestatic jaundice; Parkinson's syndrome; akathisia; dystonic reactions; inhibition of ejaculation; blood dyscrasias; photosensitivity; allergic skin reactions	Lenticular pigmentation; EGG abnormalities, usually without cardiac injury
2. Piperazine derivatives Prochlorperazine (COMPAZINE) Trifluoperazine (STELAZINE) Perphenazine (TRILAFON) Fluphenazine (PROXILIXIN; PERMITIL) Thiopropazate (DARTAL) Acetophenazine (TINDAL) Butaperazine (REPOISE) Carphenazine (PROKETAZINE)	Parkinson's syndrome; akathisia; dystonic reactions; anti-cholinergic effects	PHOTOSENSITIVITY REACTIONS: INHIBITION OF EJACULATION	Cholestatic jaundice; blood dyscrasia; lenticular pigmentation; postural hypotension; allergic skin reaction; EGG abnormalities, usually without cardiac injury.
3. Piperidine derivatives Thioridazine (MELLARIL) Mesoridazine (SERENTIL) Piperacetazine (QUIDE)	Oversedation; anticholinergic effects; postural hypotension	Pigmentary retinopathy; Parkinson's syndrome; akathisia; dystonic reactions; inhibition of ejaculation; photosensitivity reactions	Cholestatic jaundice; blood dyscrasia
B. BUTYROPHENONES Haloperidol (HALDOL) Droperidol (INAPSINE)	Parkinson's syndrome; akathisia; dystonic reactions	Blood dyscrasia; postural hypotension and tachycardia	Cholestatic jaundice; photosensitivity reaction; allergic skin reactions.
C. THIOXANTHENES Chlorprothixene (TARACTAN) Thiothixene (NAVANE)	Oversedation	Parkinson's syndrome; akathisia; dystonic reactions; postural hypontension and tachycardia; anticholinergic effects	Allergic skin reactions; blood dyscrasia; photosensitivity reaction; cholestatic jaundice

TABLE 2

COMPARISON OF THE PHARMACOLOGICAL EFFECTS
OF NEUROLEPTIC AGENTS WITH THOSE OF
THE ANXIOLYTIC SEDATIVES

A. Effects of neuroleptic agents (major tranquilizers)
   1. Produced emotional calmness and mental relaxation
   2. Highly effective in controlling symptoms of acutely and chronically disturbed psychotic patients
   3. Cause reversible extrapyramidal symptoms in susceptible patients
   4. Little to no tendency to produce physical dependence or habituation
   5. In usual doses do not depress cortex

B. Effects of anxiolytic sedatives (minor tranquilizers)
   1. Produce calmness and relaxation but not of the same "quality" as that induced by major tranquilizers
   2. DO NOT possess anti-psychotic activity of major tranquilizers
   3. Particularly effective in treatment of common psychoneurotic states such as nervous tension, mild depression, psychosomatic disorders, etc.
   4. Do not produce extrapyramidal symptoms and relatively low incidence of annoying side effects
   5. Some physical dependence may occur depending on the dose taken and duration of therapy
   6. May have some degree of cortical depression activity. This class could contain and CNS depressant drug by broad definition e.g. barbiturates
   7. Generally less effect on peripheral autonomic nervous system
   8. Some anti-convulsant properties
   9. Depressant activity on spinal reflex activity (Polysynaptic reflexes).

Table 3

Comparison of Anxiolytic Sedatives
(at anxiolytic doses)

	Benzodiazepine	Carbamates
SEDATION (Drowsiness-side effect)	Weak	Moderate
"TAMING"	Strong	Weak
ANTI-CONVULSANT	Strong	Moderate
SKELETAL MUSCLE RELAXANT	Strong-Moderate	Weak-Moderate
IMPAIRMENT OF PERFORMANCE (Ataxia)	Weak-Moderate	Moderate-Strong
ANXIOLYTIC ACTION	Strong	Moderate
BLOCK OF AGRESSIVE BEHAVIOR	Strong	Weak (without sedation) Moderate (with sedation)
PERIPHERAL AUTONOMIC NERVOUS SYSTEM	Weak (anticholinergic)	None
OVERALL TOXICITY	Moderate	Weak
TOLERANCE AND PSYCHOLOGICAL DEPENDENCE	Weak	Strong

Table 4
University of Maryland Dental School
Department of Pharmacology

DIFFERENCES BETWEEN MAO-I AND TRICYCLIC TYPE ANTIDEPRESSANT AGENTS

Type Effect	MAO-I Antidepressants	Tricyclic Antidepressants
Biogenic Amine Stores	Increase amine stores in adrenergic nerve endings and brain;	Block uptake of norepinephrine into nerve ending; decrease in intraneuronal stores of norepinephrine and 5-hydroxytryptamine; increase active amine (norepinephrine) at receptors
Autonomic Nervous System	No direct effects	Potent anticholinergic activity (anti-muscarinic) both centrally (CNS) and peripherally
Antihistaminic Activity	None	Antihistaminic
Effect of Tyramine (foods, wines, cheeses)	Increase pressor action of tyramine	Inhibit effects of tyramine by blocking its uptake into nerve ending
Effect of norepinephrine and epinephrine administered exogenously	No great alteration of peripheral effects of norepinephrine and epinephrine	Increased effects both centrally and peripherally of exogenously administered norepinephrine and epinephrine
Sedative effects	None	Sedation similar to that produced by chlorpromazine; especially prominent with imipramine and amitriptyline.

Table 5

DRUG INTERACTIONS WITH MAO-INHIBITORS

Drug	Reaction	Comment
A. Analgesics Morphine, Meperidine, Codeine, etc.	Marked potentiation of depressant effects: sedative, hypotensive, respiratory depression may cause B.P. fall, C-V collapse, respiratory failure, coma and death	May be fatal
B. CNS depressants General anesthetics Local anesthetics (systemic toxicity) Barbiturates Non-barbiturate sedatives Phenothiazine derivatives Alcohol	Depressant effects potentiated: prolonged action. Hypotension, coma	May be fatal. Many deaths reported
C. Vasopressor substances 1. All indirectly acting sympathomimetic amines e.g. Amphetamine Methamphetamine Ephedrine Phenylephrine - (partially indirect acting) Tyramine Several others	Central and peripheral effects potentiated. Marked rise in B.P., Hypertensive crises, excitement, cardiac arrhythmias, chest pain, severe headache	Intracranial bleeding, circulatory failure and death have occurred
2. Direct acting Norepinephrine Epinephrine	Peripheral effects not potentiated. Central effects enhanced	
D. Anti-hypertensives Ganglionic blockers Diuretics Guanethidine (ISMELIN)	Potentiates hypotensive effect; C-V collapse and shock	
E. Anti-cholinergics Atropine, other derivatives	Potentiates effects	
F. Others Reserpine Caffeine Insulin Corticosteroids Thiazide diuretics	Excitement, delirium, hypertension Potentiated Potentiated (Hypoglycemia) Potentiated Potentiation of CNS effects of MAO inhibitor: psychomotor stimulation, postural hypotension	

Psychopharmacologic and Analgesic Agents Employed in the Terminal Care of 78 Oral Cancer Patients

Ivan K. Goldberg*, Austin H. Kutscher**
Bernard Schoenberg*, Harvey Gralnick*** and
Harlan Kutscher****

Pharmacotherapeutics, especially psychopharmacology, plays an essential role in the manifold aspects of thanatology. Psychopharmacological agents, as well as analgesics (both narcotic and non-narcotic), are felt by many to be essential for allowing the terminal patient to die in a dignified manner. The care of terminal oral cancer patients poses particular and difficult problems because of the painful physiologic and psychological aspects of the disease, and the frequently-encountered disease-induced disfigurement as well as the required but disfiguring surgery.

The data which are reported herein are intended to depict how a competent group of physicians in a major university medical center and hospital employed psychopharmacological agents and analgesics in the management of the terminal oral cancer patient. Here, in a sense, is a report on the state of the art. At present, it represents the thinking of a group of physicians of widely disparate training, philosophy, and background, set against a framework imposed by both the care facilities and institutional demands and directives of the medical center of which they are a part. It is also intended as a baseline of information from which further studies in this general area can be better proposed.

Hopefully, these further studies will enable a set of guidelines to be established for future uses of these drugs which will bring about both the maximal medical and psychosocial well-being of the patient, and the psychological welfare of his family.

---

* Department of Psychiatry, College of Physicians and Surgeons, Columbia University, New York, New York.
** School of Dental and Oral Surgery, Columbia University, New York; Director, New York State Psychiatric Institute Dental Service, New York, New York.
*** Student, School of Dental and Oral Surgery, Columbia University, New York, New York.
**** Student, College of Physicians and Surgeons, Columbia University, New York, New York.

It is important to emphasize at the outset that this study should not be construed as an evaluation of the effectiveness of drug groups or individual drugs.

Methods

The psychopharmacologic and narcotic analgesic care of 78 patients, aged 23 to 89, 56 males and 22 females, who died of cancer in a university teaching hospital supplied the data reported herein. The study was limited to those patients who had died of cancer during the period from 1945 to 1969 in order to include only the relatively more recent modalities of psychopharmacological care. It was felt that this approach would permit the compilation of a sufficient volume of information to allow preliminary observations to be made and to develop a number of pertinent hypotheses for further study.

Based on the data obtained from their hospital charts, extensive background information sheets were completed for each of the 78 patients. A complete daily record of the drugs administered during the 21 days preceding and including the day of death was compiled for each patient. In general, the drugs pertinent to the present study—the psychopharmacologic agents and analgesics (including the narcotic analgesics)—were broken down into five categories (see below). The daily recordings included the individual dose, the route and, where clearly evident, the number of administrations per day of each drug. Total daily dosages administered could not be determined in all cases with sufficient accuracy to permit the drawing of decisive conclusions—the limit of known accuracy being set at the documented administration of the drug at least once during the course of each day included in the study.

The five drug categories utilized and involved were: antidepressant agents, antipsychotic agents, anti-anxiety agents, sedative-hypnotics and analgesics (both narcotic and non-narcotic). Special attention was also given to psychopharmacotherapy during the 24 hours prior to death.

This paper is concerned with an overall survey of the drug therapy compiled for a period of 21 days prior to death. Separate manuscripts concerned with drug use on the day of death and use of each of the drug groups studied for the final 21 days are also currently being compiled. In addition, a report in which such drug therapy is considered primarily from the viewpoint of the disease—oral cancer—is in preparation.

Results

Table I presents (to permit brevity) the percentage of patients receiving thirteen selected agents on the 21st, 14th, 7th and final day of life the patients—in which the distinctive trends are readily apparent. Results for eight drugs are not included.*

A. There was a comparative paucity of use of the minor tranquilizers (anti-anxiety agents).

Whether this represents the conclusion on the part of this staff of the ineffectiveness of such agents, or represents a lack of familiarity with the benefits ascribed to them in the European literature, is not readily apparent.

B. The use of the major tranquilizers (antipsychotic agents) is largely restricted to Thorazine (in particular) and Compazine (the latter probably for its antinausea activity). In Table I, Thorazine usage gradually climbs, and although it does not appear on the table actually reached a peak (20.8%) on the day before death, while the corresponding use of Compazine maintains a relatively constant level the week before death.

C. Both codeine and Darvon remain at a constant level, until a decreasing trend is seen during the week before death—until the day of death. It should be noted that the use of Darvon is infrequent.

D. Demerol is the most frequently employed narcotic, and its use gradually increases throughout the entire 21-day period of study.

E. The use of morphine climbs steeply as the date of death approaches, reaching a peak on the last day. It is of interest, however, that, in many instances, morphine is administered on the last day only or its administration had been begun only 2 to 3 days before the day of death. However, 14 of the 26 patients who did receive morphine received it before the 5th day prior to death.

---

* Day 1 represents the calendar date of death and, therefore, since virtually no patients lived through the entirety of that calendar date, does not represent a complete 24 hour day. Hence, in this paper, certain drugs ordered were not administered because the patient died prior to the time of day at which these drugs were to be given. The final 24 hours of drug therapy in contradistinction to the calendar day have been reported on in a paper in press in another publication.

F. Methadone was found to be used to only a minor degree by the clinicians. The use remained steady throughout almost the entire 21-day period, falling off only on the day of death.

G. The use of sedatives and hypnotics was found to climb slowly until about the last 5 days and then to taper off rather sharply.

H. Changes from lesser to more potent analgesics were common. Although aspirin, Darvon and codeine were used considerably, they were rarely the strongest analgesic employed. Demerol often replaced these 3 agents or later was given concomitantly with one of them. And Demerol itself was often succeeded by morphine.

I. The trend from Darvon or codeine to Demerol was to be expected on the basis of relief of pain. This latter changeover may, however, also have been markedly influenced by the desire of the clinician to alter reaction to pain through the introduction of a strongly euphoric *narcotic* analgesic; likewise, although the switch from Demerol to morphine was to be expected on the presumptive basis of an increase in the severity of pain, it too also might largely represent the clinician's attempt to further alter reaction to pain through the administration of the *narcotic* morphine.

J. Aspirin was found to play an extremely minor role in the management of the dying patient at any point in the last 21 days, as might be expected. Indeed, aspirin often was administered presumably primarily for its antipyretic rather than analgesic effect.

Discussion

It is reiterated that this report is specifically a review of how terminal oral cancer patients are managed at one teaching hospital by the use of psychopharmacologic agents and narcotic analgesics. Although it is recognized that the retrospective technique utilized in gathering such data presents numerous pitfalls, it should also be recognized that it has other and distinctive advantages over a prospective study in which the clinicians have knowledge of the fact that their administration of drugs is being studied by a group of investigators—and, therefore, may be concerned by the implications of monitoring, censorship, etc. Nevertheless, it is realized that a prospective study of which all hospital personnel are aware might result in different data.

It is apparent that physicians switch to morphine only with great hesitation. Morphine is well acknowledged as a more potent analgesic and narcotic than Demerol. The fact that patients are not switched from Demerol to morphine in a great many more situations suggests that many physicians feel that this drug is not essential, whereas others who do switch to morphine are persuaded that the progression is one to which the patient is entitled. If, as has been suggested, Demerol is essentially as potent a respiratory depressant as morphine, then this further reason cited in the past for not using morphine, as opposed to Demerol, should be cast aside—particularly in terminal cases. For reasons not fully explicable, there seems to be less than optimal use of antidepressant agents and the phenothiazines in the management of the terminal oral cancer patient.

Parenthetically, it should be noted that when one observes the general parallelism of the slope of the curves for Librium and Seconal, the question is raised as to whether or not this parallelism results from the use of Librium as a simple sedative.

It is noteworthy that three of the patients received no medication at any time during their last 21 days in the hospital. Whether this represents a lack of pain or a comatose state on the part of the patient, or a failure of the staff to understand the psychological and analgesic needs of the patient, cannot be commented upon in a retrospective study.

Queries Raised

The results and findings of this study pose a number of important questions for further consideration.

Among the foremost of these is the concern regarding addiction exhibited by physicians in their management of the terminal oral cancer patient. It would appear that serious study should be given to the psychological factors involved not only in relation to patient care and management, but also in relation to the concept of addiction as such in the terminal patient—and no less so in regard to the physician's emotional response to the possibility of his addicting the patient.

If phenothiazines are effective in blunting the patient's reaction to pain, one wonders why they are not employed for the benefit of a larger number of patients? Are not the clinical effects resulting in the subjective blunting of reactions to pain just as important as the blunting of the pain itself or the raising of the threshold to pain? Hence, the attributes of phenothiazines (apart from such of its effects which make possible the use of lower dosages of narcotic analgesics) should perhaps be accorded further controlled investigations under various situations of terminal care.

A major question which emerges is whether morphine may not be the most under-utilized drug of all.

Summary

This is a study of the use of psychopharmacologic agents and narcotic analgesic agents employed in the management of the terminal oral cancer patient in a major teaching hospital. The frequency and/or infrequency of the utilization of these agents is described (but not the success or failure of this approach). Distinct patterns are observable; comparatively minimal usage of certain agents is noticed; a number of questions are raised as to the proper employment of these agents, the potential in their further or improved use is considered; problems of a moral nature which might be encountered are related; the matter of addiction is discussed; anxiety concerning possible overmedication of the patient is noted; further studies to answer the quesions raised are recommended.

Footnotes (See Table I)

* It should be emphasized that not all of the patients included in a given percentage (to whom a specific drug is administered on a selected day) are the same patients to whom the drug was administered on other days. Thus, a larger total number of patients received Demerol than received it on any given day; and a patient receiving Demerol on Day 7 prior to death, thereby contributing to the percentage of patients on Demerol on that particular day, need not necessarily be the same individual who contributed to the total number (or percentage) of patients on Demerol on Day 21.

**Not all patients in the study were in the hospital for each of the last 21 days prior to their death. Therefore, the actual total number of patients on any given day (usually) was less than equal to the total number of patients (78) in the study. Hence, the actual percentage equals the number of patients receiving a drug on a given day divided by the actual number of patients (from among these 78) who were in the hospital on that particular day.

Table I*
KEY DRUGS
Total # of Pts. / Actual % of Pts.**

	DAYS			
	21	14	7	1
Demerol				
Total # Pts.	7	15	18	17
Actual % Pts.	17.1	31.9	30.0	21.8
Morphine				
Total # Pts.	3	5	7	27
Actual % Pts.	7.3	10.6	11.7	21.8
ASA				
Total # Pts.	7	9	11	5
Actual % Pts.	17.1	19.1	18.3	6.4
Codeine				
Total # Pts.	9	9	12	5
Actual % Pts.	22.0	19.1	20.0	6.4
Darvon				
Total # Pts.	5	3	5	0
Actual % Pts.	12.2	6.4	8.3	0.0
Methadone				
Total # Pts.	2	3	3	1
Actual % Pts.	4.9	6.4	5.0	1.3
Thorazine				
Total # Pts.	4	5	9	9
Actual % Pts.	9.8	10.6	15.0	11.5
Compazine				
Total # Pts.	2	3	5	1
Actual % Pts.	4.9	6.4	8.3	1.3
Librium				
Total # Pts.	2	1	3	0
Actual % Pts.	4.9	2.1	5.0	0.0
Equanil				
Total # Pts.	1	1	1	0
Actual % Pts.	2.4	2.1	1.7	0.0
Seconal				
Total # Pts.	11	12	14	9
Actual % Pts.	26.8	25.5	23.3	11.5
Phenobarbital				
Total # Pts.	5	5	8	9
Actual % Pts.	12.1	10.6	13.3	11.5
Chloral hydrate				
Total # Pts.	5	4	3	4
Actual % Pts.	12.2	8.5	5.0	5.1

Oral Care of the Terminally Ill Child

*Alben B. Curtis**

Children with an illness considered to be terminal in nature may represent a variety of conditions, each with its own unique problems. The length of survival may range from minutes in the case of the accident victim to hours in the case of acute toxic states and years in instances of cystic fibrosis and muscular dystrophy. Some children may be institutionalized throughout their terminal illness. Others may deteriorate over a long period of time with intermittent hospitalizations, and others may have periods of normalcy with a short episode of critical illness. Obviously, the oral needs for these many fatal conditions vary considerably.

Our experience in providing dental care for children with cancer, and especially leukemia, suggests that the child with a diagnosis of acute lymphocytic leukemia provides the most poignant example of a child with a terminal illness. Historically, the diagnosis of leukemia was followed by death. The use of multiple drug antineoplastic chemotherapy has produced profound changes in this once rapidly fatal disease. The chance for remission from disease is excellent; however, the length of time from the first remission of signs and symptoms of leukemia until recurrence of these cancerous cells is unknown for the individual patient—maybe weeks, maybe years, maybe never. The immunosuppressive action of the antineoplastic drugs renders the child susceptible to infections; thus, critical episodes may occur in the absence of detectable leukemia. The fear of recurrence of leukemia or a fatal infectious episode is ever present.

The initial oral condition of a child with cancer is comparable to normal children of the same age except in those few cases where the disease is manifested in the oral cavity. Once therapy is initiated, many new factors influence the oral cavity and result in special problems. Drugs used to combat cancer may produce ulcerations of the oral mucous membranes. In the absence of excellent oral hygiene, a drug-related gingivitis will develop. The oral microflora is often altered, resulting in candidiasis. When irradiation therapy involves the salivary glands, changes conducive to development of rampant caries may occur. Parents of a child with a terminal illness often become indulgent to poor

---

* St. Jude Children's Research Hospital, Memphis, Tennessee.

nutritional and oral hygiene habits, which result in further deterioration of the dentition. Thus the child with cancer may present with caries, abcessed teeth, and other routine dental problems and perhaps develop special dental problems while undergoing antineoplastic therapy for the terminal illness.

The approach to the patient must be tailored to the individual circumstances based on the diagnosis and prognosis of the particular condition. Considerations for planning dental care are: What is the current general health of the patient? Will he get better, at least temporarily, or will his condition steadily deteriorate? Does he need dental care now? What are his probable future dental needs? Can procedures be done now to prevent adverse oral problems in the last few days of life? Will dental care give emotional support to the patient, especially the teenager who is very sensitive to the reactions of the people around him? When these questions are answered, the evaluation of beneficial dental treatment can be made.

When the immediate and intermediate oral needs have been determined for a patient with a specific fatal condition, the dentist must then consider the psychological aspects of the patient. Depending on previous experiences in hospitals and offices of health professionals, the younger child may be very difficult to treat or he may have learned to accept unpleasant procedures. The adolescent and older teenager may present more difficult problems. For a period of time the teenager may be hostile and/or depressed because of his fate. He may be noncommunicative and uncooperative. On the other hand, the fact that routine reparative dentistry is considered may give him an emotional lift because of the implication that death is not just around the corner.

Communicating with the parents of the child with a fatal illness can be a very difficult task. For example, during the first few days following the diagnosis of leukemia, the parents may be in somewhat of a state of shock. It is useless to talk about oral health care for about one week following the diagnosis, except for acute existing oral problems. Many parents start a mourning process at the time of diagnosis. Some develop a "what's the use" attitude, while others receive comfort by cooperating fully with the health team's suggestions. As a consequence, the dentist may be faced with the difficult task of obtaining consent for much needed dental care for the "preterminal" child. Or he may be confronted with a barrage of questions and misinterpretations by the overly cooperative parent.

Most people in the health professions have difficulty in accepting death in the young. Avoidance and complete rejection of the child with a terminal illness are reactions often seen in those responsible for his general well-being and comfort. When the dentist refuses to provide adequate care on the basis of the diagnosis rather than the current status of the patient, a strong feeling of having been rejected may be elicited from the patient. This may result in further emotional trauma for the parents, since, in addition to his terminal illness, their child has become a social outcast.

The management of the child with cancer depends to a large degree upon the diagnosis, prognosis and methods of anticancer therapy. Some typical situations are presented and discussed below.

A 5-year-old child just begun on a treatment regime for acute lymphocytic leukemia which produces a 90 per cent one-year survival rate and a 60 per cent two-year survival rate has the oral condition described below. There is no evidence of previous dental treatment. All molar teeth exhibit carious lesions. One tooth appears to be abcessed and another has a large carious lesion with possible pulpal involvement. Oral hygiene is average for his age. A very mild gingivitis is present, but no more severe than a healthy child with similar oral hygiene. There is no complaint of oral pain.

Until there is a positive response to the antineoplastic drugs and some evidence of recovery of bone marrow, usually two to four weeks, no dental treatment should be initiated. Acute or persistent oral pain may dictate initiation of conservative therapy prior to the patient's achieving a complete remission from leukemia. Once the patient's condition has stabilized, extraction of the abcessed tooth and routine repair of the remaining teeth, including chrome steel crowns and pulpotomies where indicated, should be initiated. This is usually between four and six weeks following initiation of antineoplastic chemotherapy. During the course of dental treatment, oral hygiene techniques should be demonstrated to the parents. The necessity of good oral hygiene to reduce oral problems from drug toxicity should be stressed. Upon completion of the restorative procedures, the patient should be placed on recall and checked periodically for excellence of oral hygiene.

During a complete remission from leukemia, but while receiving maintenance drugs, the child can be managed similarly to a normal child. As long as the child is clinically healthy, and the WBC is above 2,000 with a normal differential count, the hemoglobin above 9 grams, and the platelets above 100,000^3 mm, no special precautions are required for routine dental treatment. When the laboratory values are below the above values, dental treatment should be done only when the child's physician accepts the responsibility for complications that may result.

A 13-year-old child who had a leg amputated because of osteogenic sarcoma has received antineoplastic drugs for four months and has the following oral condition at his regular six month dental recall. The anterior teeth are crowded, and the child wants to begin orthodontic therapy. Two small carious lesions are detected on radiographs. This child does not like to have his teeth filled, and has a relatively low caries attack rate.

A telephone conversation with the physician treating this child reveals that a suspicious area was seen on a recent chest film suggestive of a metastatic lesion.

Reparative dental treatment for this patient is not required. The small lesions need not be filled; however, the need for perfect oral hygiene to stop the progression of the lesion should be stressed, and a four month recall appointment given "to see if the cavities have stopped." No orthodontic therapy can be initiated for three to six months following cessation of antineoplastic therapy.

When the situation is handled in this manner, the child can leave the dental office in a positive frame of mind rather than be made to suffer through one more depressing episode prior to possible terminal hospitalization.

A child who has relapsed for the third time with acute lymphocytic leukemia, and has ulcerations of the oral mucous membranes secondary to drugs used in an attempt to induce another remission, develops profuse oozing from the oral cavity. Although the platelet content is known to be grossly inadequate and must be replaced to control bleeding, the physician attending the patient thinks the platelets may not arrive in time, unless the oral bleeding is controlled. Topical applications of 1:1,000 epinephrine and thromboplastin have been unsuccessful.

Oral manipulation alone will not completely control the bleeding in this case. The major contribution by the dentist is to isolate the bleeding sites and control the bleeding as much as possible until adequate systemic measures can be instituted. Following removal of all blood-saliva clots and after cleaning the mouth as well as possible, the dentist can determine the actual bleeding sites. Oral bandages are very useful in covering the bleeding surfaces and a gauze sponge placed over the bandage can be used to exert sufficient pressure to decrease the bleeding.

When a child has been receiving antineoplastic chemotherapy for a long period of time and has recurrent disease, his overall response becomes very unfavorable. He is very susceptible to infections; his capillaries become fragile; and his bone marrow is very depressed. Other than the situation cited above, a loose deciduous tooth might be removed in a professional office at the convenience of the dentist and physician rather than at home at night, when it might be difficult to obtain blood components necessary for control of bleeding. Dental procedures should be minimal and with specific purpose.

What Role or Roles Might the Dentist Assume in the Care of the Terminally Ill Child?

First, as a consultant the dentist may make recommendations to improve the quality of life, if not the survival time, of the child. Even in cases where he is only superficially acquainted with the therapy for the terminal illness, his knowledge of oral structures and diseases can provide significant benefits to the patient. In this role as advisor to the physician, his personal contact with the patient and parent may be minimal, but his consultation may give considerable emotional support to the parent.

Second, the dentist may see a terminally ill child at the request of the physician for emergency dental care that can be accomplished in one or two visits. This may require slightly more interaction than the consultation; however, the dentist in this position still can maintain emotional distance from the patient or the parent, if he chooses.

Third, the most frequent type of involvement probably results from a child who has been a regular dental patient and who develops a fatal disease. Such a situation is likely to produce the most emotional turmoil for the dentist who is rarely involved in the care of acutely ill or dying patients. His training and experience usually have not adequately prepared him for the treatment of terminal patients in conjunction with other health professionals. The dentist often wants to be of help but feels inadequate. He is often willing to perform technical procedures suggested by others, but is inclined to avoid making decisions himself pertaining to the oral care requirements. His personal reaction is to avoid death and dying, while his professional reaction is to do what is necessary for the health and comfort of the child.

The fourth role of the dentist in the care of the terminally ill child is found in an institutional setting. As a member of a health team, he is responsible for the oral care of patients who may have terminal illnesses.

In dealing with children with cancer at St. Jude Children's Research Hospital, Memphis, Tennessee, my own attitudes were influenced greatly by a staff experienced in the care of childhood neoplasms. A personal emotional adjustment to the reality of death in childhood was required not only of me, but of my staff. One of my staff members could not make a functional adjustment and chose to leave in spite of an intense loyalty to the patients, the institution, and to me.

Perhaps the greatest difficulty in providing care for the terminally ill child is in developing the honest interpersonal relationship necessary to win the respect of a child and yet accept the fact that this relationship may terminate rather suddenly and with finality. Nevertheless to provide the child with an optimal chance for survival and comfort, a working relationship is imperative.

If the personal emotional reaction clouds a realistic evaluation, additional unwanted stress may be placed on the dentist as well as the patient and the family. Extreme examples are refusing to extract a tooth in a child with leukemia just because of the diagnosis, rather than the ability of the patient to withstand the procedure, and subjecting the child to traumatic procedures unnecessarily because of refusal to accept impending death.

The need for professional care of the oral cavity does not end with the diagnosis of a potentially terminal illness—especially if the child may continue to live for several months or years. Yet, those having to deal with the oral problems of the dying child often can find no reference material or consultants for help in solving specific problems. Burdened with fear of doing the wrong thing with the terminal patient, many dentists withdraw completely from these patients.

The physician must assume the overall responsibility for the health and comfort of the child with a terminal illness. In those specific areas where the physician's training is limited, such as the oral cavity, it is his responsibility to seek those who are better qualified to provide treatment. The dentist must work closely with the physician to provide the oral care needed by the specific terminal patient. It is only through the combined efforts of many individuals that a dying child can live in a relatively pleasant, comfortable and rewarding environment until death.

Management of Oral Problems in the Dying Child

*Martin I. Lorin**

First, it must be recognized that the mouth is much more than simply a portal of entry for food; it is an active, multifunctional organ. The mouth is a critical organ of communication, with most of the manipulation of the vibrating air columned into recognizable sounds accomplished by the teeth, tongue, lips and palate. Of course, this role is not limited to formal speech, but also includes facial expression and primitive sounds such as laughing and crying. In our culture, kissing is used as a communicative act in greeting and parting, as well as sexually.

The mouth can be an instrument of rejection, sublimated to speech in older children and adults, but direct and uninhibited in the early years. The infant or toddler delights in spitting out food he dislikes, but just as often, seems to delight in spitting for no apparent reason. In the older child, persistant vomiting may be the physical statement of psychological rejection and in the adolescent, anorexia nervosa may serve the same symbolic role.

In a primitive sense, the mouth is an important weapon, both defensive and offensive. Impairment of capability in this area can add to feelings of weakness and vulnerability in the seriously ill patient, especially the young child in whom all primitive body functions are more directly appreciated. Young children have not yet fully sublimated this combative role to language and **speech**. Biting, as an act of aggression or expression of hostility, is not uncommon in toddlers and may persist into the third and fourth years of life, much to the dismay of the parents who in turn are more than likely to react by guilt-provoking reproaches and reprimands. To such a child oral lesions and especially oral pain can have a magical meaning and may represent punishment for the forbidden act.

Richly endowed with sensory innervation, the mouth is also an organ of gratification. Relishment of the sensation of taste, for example, seems a

---

*Babies Hospital, Columbia-Presbyterian Medical Center, New York, New York.

universal human characteristic, children being no exception. Aside from taste per se, from the sucking activities of infancy through the sexual experiences of adolescence and adulthood, the oral structures remain a source of pleasure and comfort. Thumb sucking, over-eating and smoking are common examples of attempts at self-gratification through oral stimulation, and the frequency of addiction to these is a measure of their success. Interference with these habits precipitates discomfort and anxiety. We all recognize the emotional plight of the adult who must abstain from tobacco because of sickness, but the anguish of a child who must forego thumb sucking because of oral inflammation may go unappreciated or be misunderstood. His cries are interpreted as physical pain, his frustrations as separation and his agitations as fear. The profound effects of the loss of a basic gratification achieving activity may be completely overlooked.

When weakness, pain and debilitation have restricted general motor activity, oral function may become the critical link between the dying child and his hospital environment. The child who cannot walk or get out of bed, who perhaps cannot even use a buzzer or call device, literally depends on his voice for initiating contact with those around him. If speech is painful, it must be endured; if it is impossible, the consequences are disastrous. We have all witnessed the bedridden child calling almost constantly for the nurse, as if to reassure himself that help can be summoned, that he is not abandoned or truly helpless. In such situations, with the body racked by pain and immobilized by cachexia, a favorite food may provide one of the few physical pleasures remaining.

In view of these considerations, it is obvious that those caring for the dying child must try to maintain the functional and cosmetic integrity of the oral structures for as long as is possible. Use of the mouth should be encouraged and kept as painless as possible. Every attempt must be made to keep this region clean and esthetically pleasing.

For the child with a fatal disease, not yet in the terminal stages, routine dental care and restoration are mandatory, not only to maintain self-esteem and body-image, but also to lessen the chances of a painful crisis, such as a toothache, during the critical last days. A thoroughly decayed tooth, extracted during remission when coagulation parameters are normal, will not need to be pulled as an emergency when the situation is less under control.

Parents, already overwhelmed by the financial burdens of medical care, may express concern or doubt over the decision to proceed with elective work. They should be told of the necessity of such work despite the limited outlook and assured that every effort will be made to avoid unnecessary expense and discomfort, and that only realistically indicated treatment will be done. It is essential that the dentist communicate with the physician in charge and that he indicate this to the parents, reassuring them that he is aware of the clinical situation. Some parents, too ashamed to voice concern over money at such a time, may express their anger inappropriately, accusing the dentist, for example, of causing the child unnecessary pain. Often the patient's primary physician is in a better position to deal with these feelings and to explain to the parents that financial concern is normal and realistic and not evil. The importance of open communication among all those caring for the afflicted child cannot be overemphasized.

While it is clear that ordinary dental work and routine preventive care should be performed as usual, the question of cosmetic procedure is not so simply answered. Is the child with leukemia to have extensive orthodontic treatment? Should the adolescent with advanced cystic fibrosis have his discolored and tetracycline stained teeth ground and capped? Although these decisions will generally be made by the parents, the manner in which the dentist presents his case will be crucial. The problem should not be presented in such a way as to make the parents guilty if they elect to defer such treatment. The dentist should make the parents aware of the expected cost very early in the discourse, as well as the duration of care, discomfort, and so forth. Some families may be unable to afford these treatments, but may feel compelled to proceed, once they have been suggested, either because of guilt or of need to deny the ominous prognosis. Again, conversation between the dentist and the primary physician, or an involved social worker for example, might help work out a realistic solution.

It must be understood that to decide against such cosmetic work after an actual evaluation or estimate may have terrible implications to the patient. It may confirm his suspicion that he has a fatal disease, or he may now believe death more imminent than it really is. Perhaps worst of all, it implies that he is already partly dead, less than a whole person, unworthy of the time, effort and money we would have bestowed on him had he not been doomed.

An 8-year-old child may be only too happy to defer the time and discomfort of orthodontic treatment. On the other hand, an 18-year-old may have almost as much anxiety over his stained teeth as his cystic fibrosis itself. Each case must be decided on its own merits.

In the terminal stages of disease, oral lesions are frequent and complex. Drying of oral structures is a common problem in, and source of discomfort for, the dying child. Dry tissues are painful. Lip fissures and cracks and attempts to talk or smile bring only agony. The throat is sore and swallowing a torment. The youngster may refuse to eat or drink because of pain, and a cycle is established whereby oral dehydration leads to systemic dehydration which in turn drys the oral tissues even more. To the young child the concept of enduring pain now for future benefit is untenable and all inducements to drink may fail.

Measures to prevent or correct oral dehydration are an integral part of the terminal care of any patient, including infants and children. The attending physician should maintain adequate systemic hydration, with intravenous fluids if necessary. Legitimate desires to avoid useless or heroic therapy should not be permitted to result in unnecessary pain or discomfort to the child. Frequent, small amounts of liquid, hot, warm, cool or cold, as the *patient* prefers, are most useful. Rinses with cool water are helpful in young children. Many youngsters find saline strange and nauseating, and plain water does as well. Ice chips are refreshing, often more so than sucking candies. It must be remembered that the young child often cannot handle a large piece of ice and is bothered by the extreme cold. A sliver about the size of a nickel is ideal. If the child is unable even to rinse, his lips and mouth may be swabbed with a thoroughly wetted finger or gauze. A room humidifier (cold vapor type) is useful, especially in winter. Nipples and pacifiers appear to stimulate secretion of saliva and keep the tissues moist, so long as the infant is systemically well hydrated. They are usually rejected by the infant with intraoral sores or infection.

If oxygen is administered it should be adequately humidified. With a tent, a jet or ultrasonic nebulizer is employed. With a mask or catheter, heated nebulization is preferable to the less adequate bubble humidifiers. Oxygen catheters should be situated at the anterior nares rather than the nasopharynx, and set at as low a flow rate as is commensurate with medical needs.

Oral infections, viral, bacterial and fungal, are not uncommon in children with end stage disease, especially those receiving corticosteroids or anticancer drugs. Although many of these infections may be identified by their clinical appearance, cultures should be obtained to confirm the etiological agent, whenever possible. In general, the lesions are treated as in adults, with a few restrictions. Burning, astringent and otherwise unpleasant topical medications should be avoided if at all possible. Children understand and tolerate pain less well than adults. They are more frightened and more easily upset by painful procedures and treatment, and cannot comprehend the necessity of man-made pain. Hospitalization itself is painful and traumatic; care should be taken to avoid additional stress.

Painting the oral surfaces with gentian violet is absolutely contraindicated in children. The dying child already has a shattered body image—weak and pale from leukemia, alopecic from anticancer drugs, cachetic and barrel-chested from cystic fibrosis, or yellow and bloated from biliary atresia. The grotesque purple mouth not only further damages the patient's own body-image, it may also repel loved ones, adding to the dying child's isolation. In addition, more effective, albeit more expensive, remedies are available, namely, nystatin (Mycostatin).

Some of the fatal diseases afflicting children may affect the oral structures directly. In leukemia, infiltrated, spongy gums may be so swollen as to almost cover the teeth and make chewing exceedingly painful. Hemorrhage into the gingiva or oral mucosa is common and ulcerations may result from leukemic infiltration. Enlargement of the salivary glands may occur, but fortunately is usually painless. Treatment is directed at the underlying disorder, as well as local hygiene. It should be remembered that some of the drugs used in treating leukemia can themselves cause oral lesions. For example, amethopterin (Methotrexate) commonly causes shallow, painful ulcerations of the buccal mucosa and tongue.

Children dying from the lung destruction of cystic fibrosis may be afflicted by a variety of oral maladies. Respiratory distress, tachypnea and mouth breathing, common in the terminal stages of this disease, cause severe drying of the lips and mouth, often aggravated by the administration of oxygen. Painful, inflammatory fissures of the lips occur and are usually related to aerosol medication rather than nutritional disturbances. Temporarily substituting pancreatic nuclease (Dornavac) for acetylcysteine (Respaire, Mucomyst) or changing antibiotics may effect prompt resolution. Use of a mouthpiece rather than mask to deliver the aerosol will lessen contact of the aerosol with the lips and a simple bland ointment (petrolatum or Chap Stick) offers protection and relief.

Chronic renal disease may be associated with uremic stomatitis and ulcerative gingivitis. The solid cancers of childhood, neuroblastoma for example, may metastasize the jaw and ulcerate into the oral cavity. Certain immunological deficiencies may be associated with intractable oral moniliasis refractory to all therapy. Gentle removing of the exudate with 3% hydrogen peroxide followed by the application of a double strength solution of nystatin (200,00, n/cc) may lessen the lesions and afford some measure of relief. Infants dying with severe congenital malformations, i.e., cardiac, renal, may have an associated cleft palate that requires special care in feeding and the use of a cleft palate nipple. Solids are introduced slowly.

In summary, it should be emphasized that although we cannot cure, we can treat, and *we treat the child not the lesion.* Our therapeutic armamentarium may become exhausted, but never our interest, attention or compassion. Always, when dealing with the dying, but most especially with children, we must be gentle and cause no unnecessary pain or fear.

Dentistry and the Dying Patient
*Paul Scheman**

During chronic mortal illness or following severe acute illness or severe accidents resulting ultimately in the death of the patient, many patients require the services of the dentist or the oral surgeon. The dentist who deals with the dying patient must be a mature individual who has personally faced and dealt with the problem of his own death and the death of loved ones. If he has not come to grips with the deep philosophical and emotional questions which death raises, he cannot cope with the patient's problem. He is instead faced with an acute situation: he must address himself to these complex and disturbing questions, and the uncertainty of his reactions will be transmitted detrimentally to the dying patient. The mature dentist who *has* resolved these problems and *can* function adequately and properly in this situation should be able to share his attitudes with the intern or resident who may lack sufficient maturity to enter into a relationship with a dying patient which will not be filled with disturbing reactions for all involved.

The Role of the Dentist

The request for dental care for a dying patient with an acute clinical problem usually is directed to the oral surgeon. In most instances, this places him in a position of secondary importance to a larger surgical team. It is his responsibility to determine how important his services are in the total picture, and on that basis to determine whether or not he should perform them at all. Of course no such hesitation should occur if there is the slightest possibility that his contribution will help to avert death. If death is certain and if the injury to the face is of a mutilating character, the dentist must consider the impact of badly displaced and lacerated tissues upon the family. Although morticians have great skills in repairing a mangled and disfigured face, in many instances the prior services of a dentist can add a significant and important contribution. The repair of broken dentures is an example of such a service.

For the chronically ill patient, the coming of death is a matter of time. His dental problem presents greater complexity; however, its solution consists of adherence to basic principles. The dying patient who is not comatose is engaged in a constant struggle against the handicaps of failing functions. One of the first functions to fail is salivary secretion. This produces a state of discomfort resulting from xerostomia which makes every oral movement, including repeated involuntary swallowing, an

---

* Director of the Department of Dentistry, The Kingsbrook Jewish Medical Center, Brooklyn, New York.

unpleasant and even difficult event. The dentist must supervise and assure adequate provision for the management of oral hygiene, principally directed toward maintaining a high level of moisture in the mouth. The use of cosmetic mouth washes can result in a decrease in bacterial growth, a decrease in oral fetor, and in consequence help to make it more pleasant for those who administer nursing care and for the family.

Many patients with chronic terminal illness have been long-time full denture wearers. If possible, these dentures should not be taken from the patient. The loss of oral facial tone in the dying patient requires the support which dentures afford in order to make breathing and swallowing easier and to improve appearance. There is nothing more distressing to those in the room and to the patient than the stertor which is produced by a collapse of tissues around the oral cavity. Certainly this places a burden upon nursing care because most nurses and nurses' aides receive a non-dental type of training in the care of the oral cavity. The obvious responsibility for the hospital dentist is to institute programs in the training of nurses and auxiliaries that will make this kind of care as easy to perform as many equally unpleasant and even arduous nursing chores. As simple a procedure as frequent removal of dentures (once every two hours), rinsing them in cold or even iced water, and replacing them will render an appreciated service and improve the emotional tone of the dying patient. Also the very active care in an area as psychologically dynamic as the oral cavity will represent a non-verbal communication of tenderness which is the first and most basic principle in the dental care of the dying patient.

Other problems which the dentist will be asked to deal with are the presence of some acute infection, a broken tooth with sharp edges, or a severely mobile tooth which does not permit even minimal oral function. In these cases, usual treatment plan concepts must be set aside, even if so doing appears to violate accepted practices; the basic principle is that a specific treatment plan must be secondary to patient comfort. For example, it is far better to cover a broken tooth with a crown form without extensive excavation than to involve the patient in the grinding and preparation that would be required to place even a temporary filling. (If a denture tooth is loose, it should be extracted and replaced immediately, since the work required to replace the missing tooth is done out of the patient's mouth.) Mature judgment and ingenuity are required to determine the best plan of treatment.

The most difficult area of management of a dying patient occurs in the cancerous diseases which involve the oral cavity. The mucosal covering of the soft tissues or of the bone is destroyed and areas of varying sizes are exposed to irritation, resulting in severe pain. The same basic principle is applied to these diseases and is derived from the fact that large quantities (500 mm to 1000 mm) of irrigant solution will bring about, by dilution, a significant reduction of the bacterial flora and secondarily a decrease in pain. Through adverse osmolarity, saline or even hypotonic solutions such as warm water will also reduce the functional ability and hence the sensitivity of nerves. In many instances the application of vital dyes such as gentian violet to an open lesion for three minutes will reduce the sensitivity. The application of cortisone in an adhesive is also useful in inflamed condition brought about by chemotherapy or radiation therapy. In many of these patients the problem is essentially one of controlling odor, exudation and drooling. Odor is controlled primarily by volume irrigations as described above, but also through the use of nonalcoholic solutions of detergent mouth washes. For those patients who can do so, frequent use of flavored troches is very helpful. The problem of exudates is extremely difficult to deal with and whenever possible one should attempt to produce a temporary eschar in order to reduce the volume of fluid. The application of tannic acid powder, provided it does not gain access to the oral cavity proper, and petrolatum dressings covered with a waterproof outer covering, will keep bed clothes from staining and contribute to the patient's comfort.

The control of drooling resulting from excessive salivation is more difficult to manage. However, antisialagogues such as atropine and derivatives of atropine may be used in dosages which will reduce but not inhibit salivary flow. A drug such as Banthine may be used in this connection. Ingenuity will be needed to provide ways of retaining saliva in the oral cavity through appliances or using bibs and receptacles to collect the saliva in order to keep the bib dry and comfortable. A great deal of work needs to be done in this area since there are not too many very satisfactory answers to the problem.

Problems of the Elderly Patient

The dying elderly patient represents a special problem. Such patients fall into two broad categories: those who are fearful of dying, and who have not in their lifetime come to grips with the idea of their own death; and those who have prepared themselves for the end of their lives and accept the outcome calmly. The elderly, dying patients who are prepared for death do not present a problem to the dentist. Indeed, from these patients the dentist will learn almost all he needs to know about the way a human being should face death. It is from these wonderful people that one learns that death is merely another aspect of life. If there is any problem at all for the dentist with these patients, it is that he will find many and even trivial excuses to visit them often, at the expense of other patients who need his services more. Immature members of the house staff should be exposed to such patients rather than to the fearful elderly. Even though all the positive values may still not be appreciated by an immature individual, it will help in the resolution of his own fears and in the establishment of his own philosophical grasp as the lesson of the accepting elderly patient is communicated.

The fearful elderly patient is in need of dental care directed toward continued encouragement. These patients will seek advice, counsel and reassurance from the dentist. The fact that he is a professional, even though not involved in a life and death decision from the patient's point of view, places him in the position of a counselor. While not being directly responsible for the patient's medical management, he is presumed to have access to the chart, to the facts, to the patient's medical management, and to the patient's physician; what he says will be taken by the patient to be an accurate reflection of the state of affairs. The dentist must be careful, therefore, to advance the general program of helping the patient through the difficult and agonizing period of dying.

The Dentist and Dying Children

The chief area of concern for the dentist is in the management of the dental problems of the cancer diseases of childhood, especially leukemia. Although the life plan of these patients is as yet severely circumscribed by their disease, remissions of many years have been achieved by the newer combinations of therapies. The longer life expectancy means that the dentist will have an opportunity to do all of the needed dentistry for these patients. In the hospital, the management of leukemia cases is greatly simplified and is divided into three stages. In the first, the admission stage of the disease, little should be done other than control of pain due to severe caries. Root canal therapy and periodontal treatment and/or surgery no matter how minor, other than a careful superficial prophylaxis, is absolutely contraindicated. This acute stage may last and even be exacerbated in the course of some therapeutic modalities such as methotrexate; the end point for therapy with this drug is the appearance of oral gingival necrosis. The oral mucosa is an endodermal tissue and as such it has, as does the mucosa of the gut, a short generation time; and since the effect of many of these antimetabolites is upon the mitotic event, both of these tissues become necrotic. Following the same principle applicable during the acute admission stage, use of the water pic at low pressures as therapeutic periodontal care can now be instituted.

In the second or remission stage, all types of dentistry except those which require prolonged fatiguing sessions or extensive surgery are permitted. In the final or complete remission stage, there are no limitations on dental care.

The management of these children must be based on principles which derive from optimism for a life of normal duration. The patient should be managed on a level of interpersonal communication that reinforces this optimism; overprotectiveness should be avoided. This will serve in good stead if the remission should be prematurely terminated. There is no substitute for the rapport that results from a warm, interpersonal, protecting relationship.

Conclusion

As the dentist increases the frequency of his contacts with hospitalized patients, there will be a greater probability that he will have to face the question of death in his treatment of patients. He will do so successfully if he establishes his own sound philosophical and emotional base and thereafter uses as much ingenuity as he can muster. Life and death concern not only the dying person involved; they also become central and primary concerns for the living.

Dental Care for the Terminally Ill Patient

M. B. Quigley* and I. L. Shannon*

The need for care of the mouth and associated structures of the chronically ill or dying patient should be discussed from several points of view.

1. *The Patient.* Even though the patient is approaching death, the physiologic and pathologic processes in the oral cavity do not stop, but may in fact be exaggerated or exacerbated by such factors as drug treatment, a liquid diet, or intravenous rather than per os feeding.

An example of this was a 46-year-old woman, dying from metastatic mammary carcinoma approximately three years following radical mastectomy. She had always practiced good oral hygiene and had taken excellent care of her teeth. Some three weeks prior to her demise, the patient's chief complaint was toothache. Considerable radiation had been used and salivary gland function, particularly that of the parotids bilaterally, was greatly impared. Gingival recession had occurred and exposed root dentin was extremely sensitive on eating and brushing. The patient insisted on continuing brushing, no doubt motivated by lifelong habit.

2. *The Family.* The terminal period is a trying time when loved ones must watch a patient slowly die. Any effort to add to the patient's physical comfort is much appreciated. Remaining close to the patient will be made considerably more pleasant if the patient's oral hygiene is adequately maintained. Family mumbers might perform some of the necessary hygienic procedures and be given the feeling of participation in the welfare of the patient during these stressful days.

3. *Others.* The nursing and attending staff, friends, chaplains and others who may visit the patient are also more comfortable if the patient's oral hygiene is optimal.

What Can Be Done?

When the patient can still perform the task of brushing his teeth, he should be encouraged to do so. Obviously, if the patient is still ambulatory or can be taken by wheelchair to a washbasin, this produces no problem. Only encouragement and making certain that toothbrushes and paste are

---

* Oral Physiology Research Laboratory, Veterans Administration Hospital and The University of Texas Dental Branch, Houston, Texas.

always available are necessary. Artificial dentures should be scrupulously cleaned, and the patient should be encouraged to wear them if this is possible physiologically. Some patients will lose considerable weight in a terminal illness and bone and flesh loss in the oral regions may eventually reduce the retention of the dentures and render them useless and possibly hazardous. However, the patient should be encouraged to use them, aided by denture adhesive if necessary.

The time may arrive, however, when the patient is unable to carry out effective procedures for himself. This is no excuse for neglecting oral hygiene. The Veterans Administration Dental Service has realistically faced the problem of oral hygiene for the total nursing care patients, and has produced a film for use in training nurses and ancillary personnel in the management of the comatose and paraplegic patient (1). The techniques are based on the formulation of an ingestible toothpaste. A similar toothpaste was used by the Apollo crews during flight and even on the lunar surface. The astronauts reported that, aside from the actual oral hygiene benefits of using the ingestible dentifrice, there is a tremendous psychological lift from the use of this paste. The astronauts become uncomfortable after several days in their flight module. Bedridden patients have similar problems because of the compromised general hygiene problem. Any procedure that contributes materially to the psychologic state of the patient (particularly the dying patient) is extremely useful.

The techniques described and illustrated below are essentially those devised and depicted by the V. A. film.

Materials and Methods

The availability of ingestible toothpaste, which prevents gagging and nausea and eliminates the necessity of constant spitting, not only of the toothpaste but also of the rinse water, makes the task of cleaning the mouth and teeth much simpler. Another modern appliance which is available is the battery-driven toothbrush with changeable heads. This toothbrush has an intrinsic motion so that the person cleaning the teeth holds the brush against the surface of the tooth to be cleaned and the brush will automatically carry out the correct movements. Also available is a 0.4% stannous fluoride gel which can be applied to the teeth after each cleansing procedure. If there are areas which cannot be cleaned, a high speed water spray may be used. However, this requires an efficient vacuum aspirator, especially in the case of a recumbent patient. Directions for the care of hospitalized patients will be given first, followed by modifications which may be necessary for the home care patient.

The Hospitalized or Nursing Home Patient

The necessary equipment is assembled on a bedside tray. In the front row, from left to right, are: basin, fluoride gel, ingestible toothpaste, cotton tipped applicator, two tongue swabs, padded tongue blade for use as lip and cheek retractor, drinking straw, extra cotton applicator and extra tongue blade. In the back row, left to right, are a disposable drinking cup and electric toothbrush. Below the brush is a rubber bite block. Since the brushing procedure is somewhat lengthy, the rubber bite block may be used to keep the mouth open, and also to prevent the patient's muscles from tiring. It should be noted that the padded tongue depressor is used to retract the cheek, lip and tongue when the buccal and lingual surfaces of the teeth and gingivae are being cleaned. The occlusal surface must receive separate attention. A standardized routine should be followed. One quadrant of the mouth should be completed at a time. The nurse or other personnel may use a suction apparatus to remove excess water and saliva which may collect in the floor of the mouth. On completion of rinsing, all the surfaces of the teeth may be coated with the stannous fluoride gel applied with cotton. The surface of the tongue may be gently cleaned with a soft brush or sponges.

If the nurse cleans an artificial denture, this should be done over a bowl of water, so that if the denture should slip accidentally from the hand, breaking and chipping will be minimal. As was pointed out previously, dentures may become loose due to cachexia. If denture adhesive is being used, it should be removed thoroughly at each cleaning before more adhesive is applied.

The Patient at Home

All of the above procedures can be carried out at home. If the patient is able to sit up in bed, an emesis basin or similar receptacle can be held under his chin and excess fluid allowed to drain. In the prone patient this presents a problem and some hand-held mechanical aspirator must be used if extensive rinsing of the mouth is to be carried out. However, even if the aspirator is not available, the ingestible toothpaste can still be used.

Other Problems

As mentioned earlier, in the case of gingival resorption, pain from the exposed dentin of the root becomes a major problem. A desensitizing toothpaste (several are available on the market) has proved effective in substantially reducing the patient's discomfort, and encouraging the patient to eat. Even the family benefits from this, knowing that at least some of the patient's suffering has been ameliorated. It has been shown that the 0.4 stannous fluoride gel will also reduce dentin sensitivity (2).

Daily topical applications of fluoride gel, either brushed onto the teeth or by application in a mouthguard type of appliance, are now being used in Veterans Administration Hospitals to minimize caries in postradiation patients with impaired salivary flow. In this way osteoradionecrosis, which so often follows extraction of teeth in these patients, will be minimized.

Obviously, routine dental care such as permanent restorations will not be undertaken, but all painful and uncomfortable dental conditions must be taken care of, even if the treatment is only palliative. Routine extraction of loose painful abscessed teeth also may be considered. No one need suffer dental pain, even those patients who are terminally ill. With the proper consultations between physician and dentist, and physician, dentist and family, all that can should be done to prevent the patient from suffering needlessly.

References

1. This film is available on loan from Dental Training Center, Veterans Administration Hospital, 50 Irving Street, N. W., Washington, D. C., 20422

2. J. T. Miller, I. L. Shannon, W. E. Kilgore, and R. H. Bookman, "Use of a Waterfree Stannous Fluoride Containing Gel in the Control of Dental Hypersensitivity," *Journal of Periodontology,* 40 (8):491, 1969

Acknowledgments

The authors wish to thank Mrs. Godwin, R.N., Mrs. Canally, R.N., and J. Morrow, D.Ds. for their help and cooperation. The assistance of the Medical Illustrations Department of the Veterans Administration Hospital, Houston, Texas, is also gratefully acknowledged.

Legends

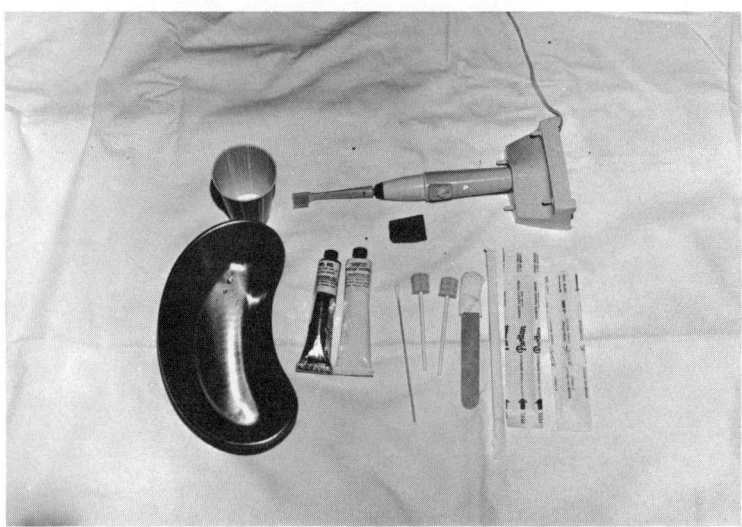

Figure 1. Bedside table equipment. *Front row, from left to right:* basin, fluoride gel, ingestible toothpaste, cotton tipped applicator, 2 tongue swabs, padded tongue blade for use as lip and cheek retractor, drinking straw, extra cotton applicator and extra tongue blade. *Back row, left to right:* disposable drinking cup and electric toothbrush. Below the brush is a rubber bite block.

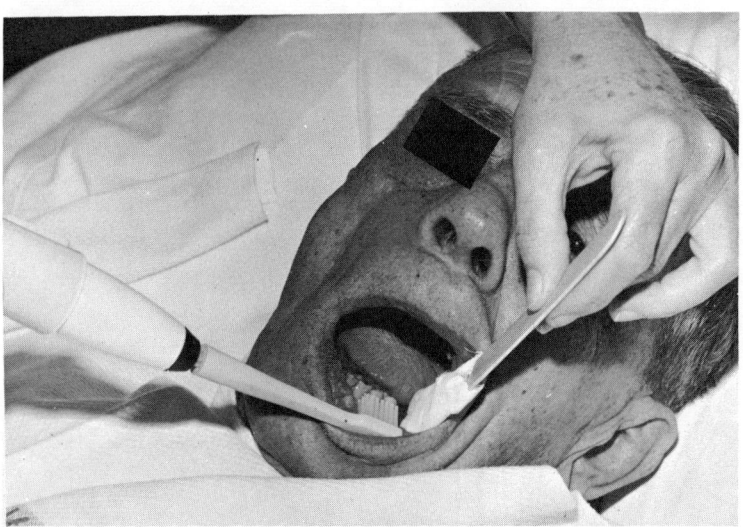

Figure 2. Buccal surfaces of lower teeth are cleaned. The padded tongue blade retracts the cheek and lips. The occlusal surfaces are cleaned separately.

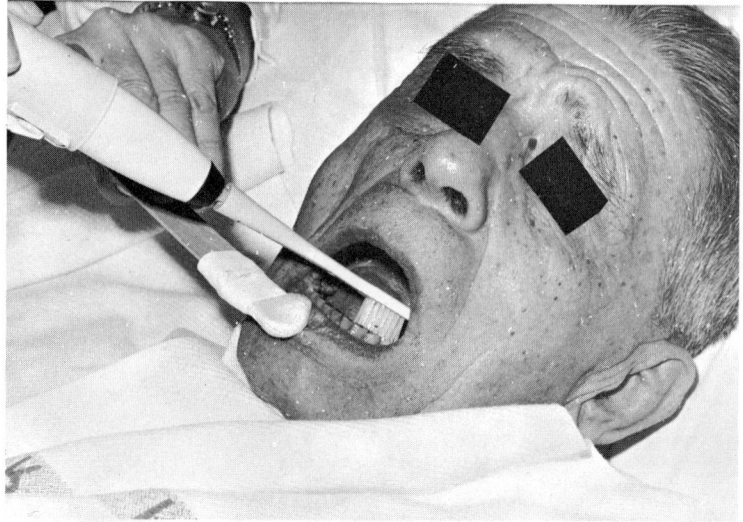

Figure 3. Application of stannous fluoride gel as the last step in the procedure.

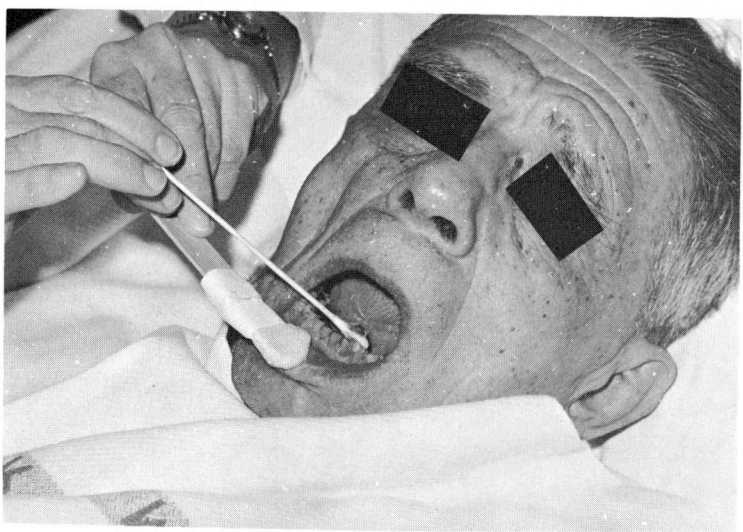

Figure 4. Artificial denture is scrubbed over a basin of water. Should the denture accidentally fall, the water will minimize chipping and breaking.

Maxillofacial Prosthesis

Norman G. Schaaf *

By definition, the maxillofacial prosthodontist is concerned with the prosthetic reconstruction and rehabilitation of the patient with a defect of the head and neck area. The anatomic defect may be present as a result of surgical intervention, congenital anomaly, or trauma. The contact of the prosthodontist with the dying is most commonly with the surgical or cancer patient.

The treatment of the cancer patient is usually in the form of surgery and/or radiation therapy. Chemosurgery, cryosurgery, and chemotherapy have also been added to the profession's armanentarium. Often we are confronted with a patient who has a significant, debilitating defect of the head and neck area but is known to have untreatable recurrent, residual or new disease. Six factors relating to the role of maxillofacial prosthetics in the care of the terminal patient should be considered.

To Provide Treatment or Not

First, no matter what the predicted life expectancy of the patient, prosthodontic care must be provided to improve his well-being.

Additional surgery is usually not necessary. The necessary procedures and treatment can be carried out without particular strain on the patient whether he is in a hospital bed, wheelchair, at home or in a hospital clinic. The fact that the person is ill is not a reason for deferring prosthodontic services.

Second, none of the treatment provided at this time is ever of a permanent nature. Two main reasons compel the construction of temporary prostheses in almost every instance. On one hand the prosthodontist is faced with the patient whose anatomical defect is continually changing, particularly soon after surgery, so that new prostheses must be provided every few months or at least every year or two. On the other hand, the materials used in this work are still less than ideal particularly because of the fact they eventually deteriorate. No matter if polyvinyl chloride, soft acrylic or silicone rubber is used for the prosthesis, it must be constructed anew every six to twelve months because

---

* Chief, Dental and Maxillofacial Prosthetic Services, Roswell Park Memorial Institute, Buffalo, New York

of the breakdown of the material. However, this is of relatively minor significance. This technique, in addition to providing several prostheses for well patients over many years, can also serve the terminal patient for the brief period of life remaining.

Third, the head-and-neck cancer patient largely falls into the fifth to eighth decade in terms of age group. The life expectancy of any individual, although relatively unknown at any point, is a basic factor in the decision whether to provide treatment or not. It is not unusual to see an apparently cured and healthy patient die of a cerebral vascular accident or myocardial infarction after the completion of extensive prosthodontic services. On the other hand, patients for whom oral or facial prostheses are constructed frequently have residual or recurrent carcinoma over a period of four or five years. If the patient can benefit from a prosthesis and is expected to live through the time needed to prepare it, the prosthodontic service should be rendered.

Fourth, the patient can often function better with a prosthesis, be more comfortable and require less care. For example, a patient who has undergone a sub-total maxillectomy requires the introduction of a nasogastric tube and a special diet in order to take in nourishment. The completion of a maxillary obturator prosthesis which separates the nasal and antral cavities from the oral cavity and restores palatal form will allow the patient to eat and speak normally. The maxillofacial prosthetic treatment thus provided can allow the patient to be removed from the hospital or extended care facility and remain at home for the remainder of his life.

Fifth, an improvement in the appearance of the patient with a facial defect can make life more pleasant both for him and those close to him. The patient who is with disease is usually not considered for surgical reconstruction and may be left with an orbital defect, loss of the nose and another area of the face. Dressings and bandages about the face are difficult to place and do not satisfy esthetic requirements. Conversely, a facial prosthesis can make the patient appear normal so he may carry on his activities without drawing needless attention. New techniques and materials, such as the use of silicone rubber in dental plaster or stone molds, can make the prosthesis available to the patient in a few hours in certain circumstances.

Sixth, the prospect of the terminal patient bearing additional costs for treatment which is not directed at the disease itself becomes a matter of conscience for the health professional. Certainly in the same vein as the surgeon who does palliative surgery even if he cannot cure the patient, prostheses must be provided for the seriously ill patient to improve his well-being. The development of governmental funding programs in some instances allows the dentist to treat the patient without increasing his financial burden. Recent government grants have supported several regional centers around the country where services of this type are available. Also, since many of the patients discussed are in-patients in hospitals, maxillofacial prosthetic treatment can be provided through the hospital dental service.

In hospital clinics and private offices the prosthodontist is occasionally confronted by patients with an illness which will cause death in a variable length of time. If the patient has a defect of the head and neck area, the maxillofacial prosthodontist has a continuing responsibility. This responsibility is to the patient and everyone caring for him. If improvement can be made in the functions of mastication, speech and/or appearance, the dentist bears the responsibility for enhancing the well-being of this patient. The imminence of the patient's death does not excuse ignoring the possibility of service to him here and now.

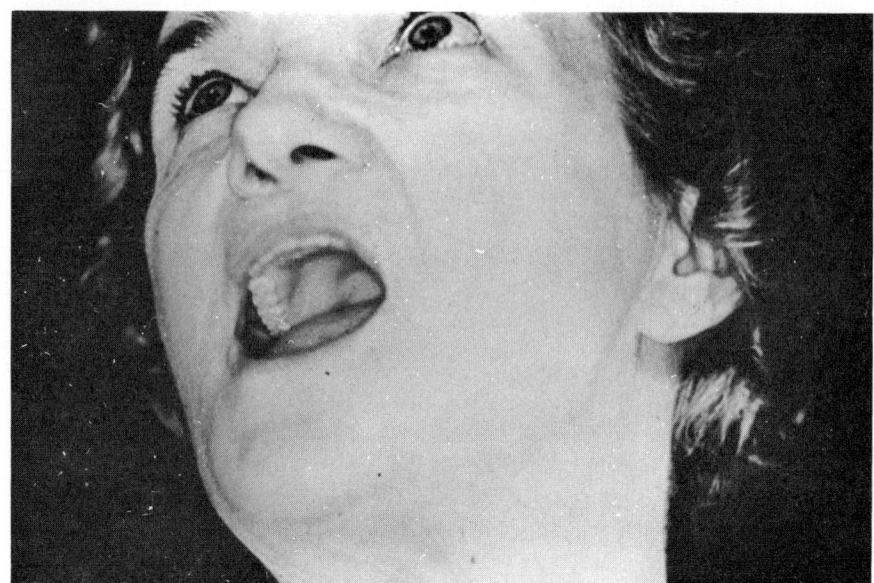

Figure 1. A large maxillary defect will not allow the patient to eat or speak normally.

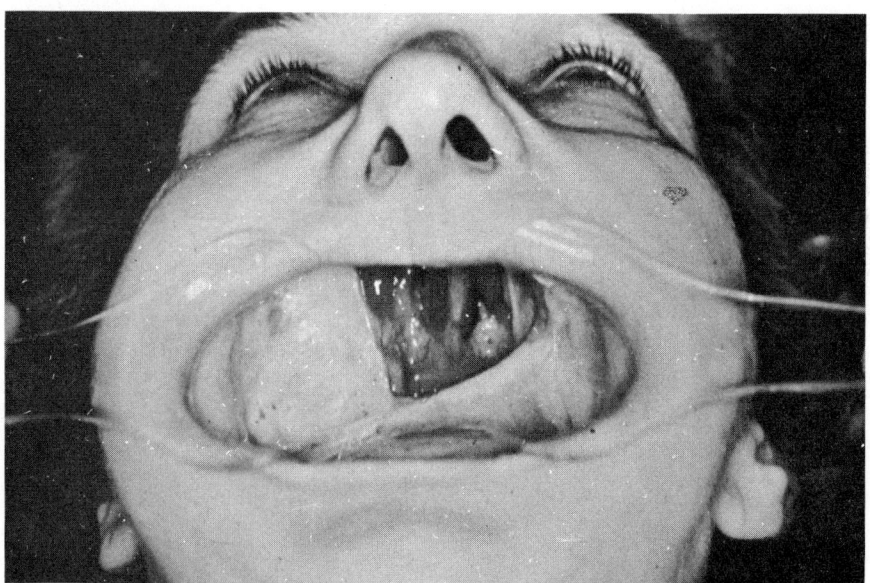

Figure 2. The placement of a prosthesis which restores normal contour and separates the oral and nasal cavities allows the patient to function normally.

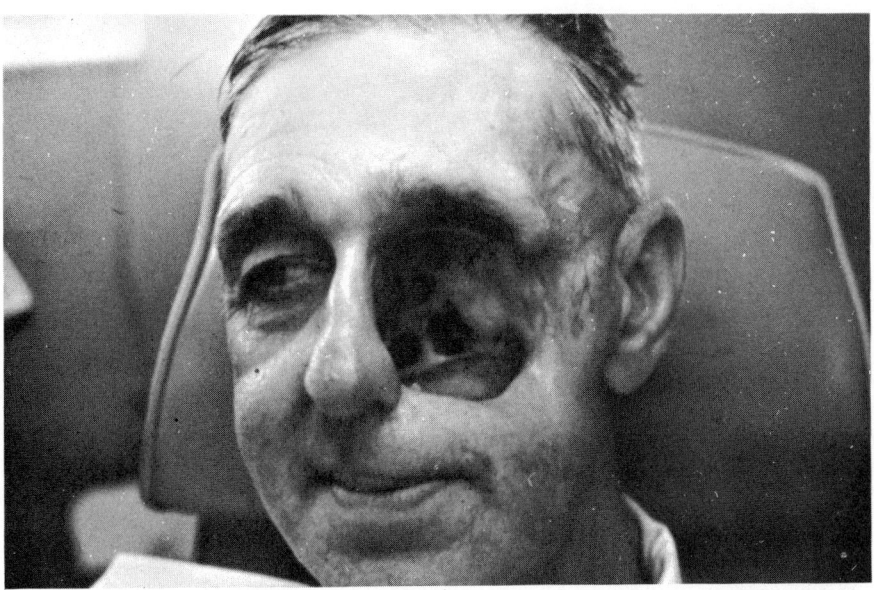

Figure 3. A large facial defect, which is difficult to dress, presents an unesthetic appearance.

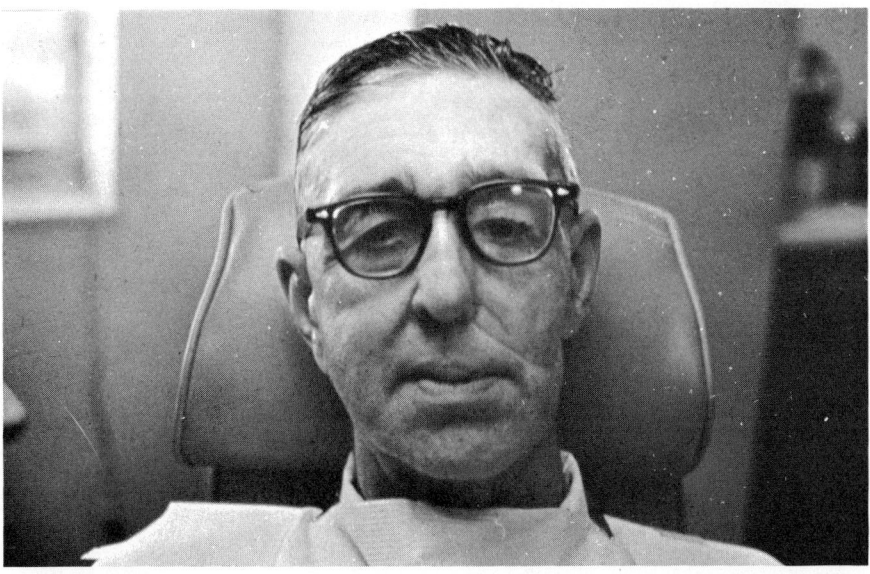

Figure 4. A facial prosthesis allows the patient to appear normal and thus function in public.

Dental Care of the Dying Patient

Clifton O. Dummett [*]

Introduction

It may be that the dental profession has exhibited little concern about mortally sick patients because dentistry is usually practiced on a relatively well, ambulatory patient. Dentists have been inclined to transfer the total responsibility for patient care to the physician once it became obvious that the possibility of death was imminent. This latter concept has not been affected by any revolutionary changes during the past thirty years.

The Hospital Defined

It used to be customary for people to die in their own homes. Then came a time when hospitals were regarded as the institutions where patients were placed to die. After all else had failed and confused medical practitioners had exhausted their sources of scientific cure, patients were sent to hospitals to await the inevitable. Today the Council on Medical Education defines a hospital as an "institution suitably located, constructed, organized, managed and personneled to supply—scientifically, economically, efficiently and without hindrance—all or any recognized part of the complex requirements for the prevention, diagnosis and treatment of physical, mental and the medical aspect of social ills; with functioning facilities for training new workers in the many special professional, technical and economic fields essential to the discharge of its proper functions; and with adequate contact with physicians, other hospitals, medical schools and all accredited health agencies engaged in the better health programs."

A currently accepted concept of modern dentistry is one which defines it as an integral part of medicine, primarily concerned with the illnesses affecting the oral cavity, its contents and associated parts. This concern embraces not only the care of healthy tissues, but also the diagnosis and therapy of pathological conditions affecting them, and in addition, the biomechanical restoration of imperfections or missing structures. These functions have become more intricate through the years, and presently, highly trained practitioners and specialties are necessary in order to carry

---

[*] Professor and Chairman, Department of Community Dentistry, University of Southern California, Los Angeles, California.

out efficient services. It is essential to keep in mind the rather comprehensive statement describing what a hospital is and what its functionings involve, while discussing the subject of oral care of patients in terminal illness. Actually, it is in the hospital setting that dentists are most likely to become involved with very sick patients.

Oral Care

The concept of "oral care" is an all-inclusive one, embracing both therapy and solicitude. This author defines oral care as the diagnosis, prevention and treatment of oral disease and disability, with a concomitant expression of a conscious concern on the part of the therapist for the anxiety, pain and suffering of the patient in question, and of his or her immediate family.

Much of the fear of dentists has emanated from a general feeling that dentists were somehow indifferent to the pain experienced by their patients. Even though many of the criticisms of indifference were over-exaggerated, there was a time, for instance, when the administration of a local anesthetic for cavity preparation was generally frowned upon, because the "pain reaction was an indication to the operator that he had reached the dento-enamel junction, and so should be aware of pulpal proximity."

Clinical Services Rendered

Oral care of patients in terminal illness consists of much dental intervention, but even more of conscious concern. In the case of the former, the most important function which can be instituted is the maintenance of some degree of oral hygiene and comfort.

In the hospital setting, with patients either in intensive care units, or under conditions of total physical disability, the functions of oral comfort and hygiene are accomplished by nurse, aide, dental hygienist, and dentist all working cooperatively, and coordinating dento-oral procedures within the general medical treatment plan.

Periodontics and endodontics are the most frequently called-upon specialties in extensively disabling circumstances. The relative inability of patients to use the oral structures properly, combined with the soft dietary regimen, the lowered tissue resistance and general oral stagnation—all are factors which promote greater susceptibility to infection, ulceration, pain and oral fetor. The success of instituting periodontal procedures is dependent upon the extensiveness of the procedures and the patient's condition, so that very often periodontic treatment may have to be limited to oral irrigation, periodontal hydrotherapy, and those phases of oral medical therapeutics which involve the application of and swabbing with medicaments.

Exodontia and minor oral surgery will be necessary when there is pain from extensive dental decay and abscesses. Such procedures must be carefully evaluated in view of the patient's condition, and the utmost care exercised if and when procedures become mandatory.

Major oral surgery is a clinical service which requires very special considerations and consultations. Much depends upon whether it is to be performed on a critically ill person, or if a patient becomes critically ill as a result of extensive oral surgery.

Restorative dentistry is another oral health service deserving consideration. In the severely ill patient, palliative procedures are advocated. The most humane procedure would be the placing of temporary restorations following the removal of as much carious material as possible. Great care should be exercised to avoid subjecting patients to the personal rigors which many restorative dental procedures require.

Insofar as prosthodontics is concerned, the primary services rendered would include cleaning, polishing, and adjusting prosthetic appliances. Replacing defective teeth and clasps of dentures are additional operations which may be accomplished.

Care of the oral soft tissues and oral comfort are, however, the most important considerations. Involved are the removal of debris, soft tissue massage, treatment of minor ulcerations, lacerations and abrasions, and the maintenance of scrupulous cleanliness of the oral cavity.

There are also clinical services which the dental department of the hospital is called upon to render after the patient has died. These include the insertion of dentures in recently deceased patients. If the dentures cannot be immediately located, there are special difficulties associated with carrying out these procedures after rigor mortis sets in.

The author recalls an unusual case in which an emergency set of dentures had to be constructed by the hospital's prosthodontist for a deceased patient. In another instance dentures had to be forcefully inserted long after the patient had succumbed, because the family insisted upon the achievement of some semblance of a suitably life-like facial appearance.

It is the responsibility of the dental department to be conversant with the status of seriously ill patients, so that clinicians would be informed as soon as death occurs, and thus be able to carry out any needed procedures. The deceased's appearance is apparently important to the surviving family. It is influenced by custom, religion and other circumstances which probably constitute the reasons why so much time, effort and money are spent in efforts to camouflage death with cosmetics, flowers, dentures and other paraphernalia.

Community Dentistry's Contributions

Community dentistry combines the elements of technical proficiency, the biological sciences and social sensitivity. It comprises that facet of a health profession engaged in providing those skills to dentists and dental auxiliaries which will enable them to be socially sensitized, scientific practitioners on an interacting population of varied individuals with common interests living in a particular area. To be socially sensitive, dentists must be able to adhere to the maxim of treating patients rather than teeth. They must also accept the ethic that all clinical procedures should be influenced by the ideal of retaining the natural dentition for life.

Like the physician in community medicine, the dentist is being called upon to regard the patient in his total environment rather than merely in terms of his dental complaint. Assistance in modifying that environment, whenever necessary, is an important additional function of the medical team of which the dentist is an integral member. As long as the dentist sincerely believes that he must work as a part of a team of trained health workers, then it is possible to institute the aforementioned environmental changes. Community dentistry is prepared to render substantive contributions to this facet of the oral care of terminal patients.

Communicating with the families of terminal patients is no more the sole responsibility of the nurse or physician or minister than is health the special domain of the medical doctor alone. The particular health professional member to whom the patient or his family relates is a much more valued contact than was formerly believed. The number of cases in which excellent rapport has been achieved between patient and dentist is significantly large, and would suggest the exploration of just what solace could be rendered and empathy achieved under dire conditions.

Because there have been significant qualitative changes in the kinds of general medical and surgical care which critically ill patients have been receiving over the past ten years, it is estimated that there has been a significant reduction in mortality rates. By and large, technological advances in equipment and sophisticated instrumentation have made these reductions possible. But much of the improvement has been due to the medical, nursing and other health personnel to whom a large share of monitoring responsibilities has been delegated. The general and specialized intensive care units in hospitals which have facilitated the grouping of very ill patients in specially designed and fully equipped areas, continuously under nursing observation and care, are well known. It is in these areas too that there has been experimentation with the use of auxiliary personnel, and the spectacular results obtained have convinced administrators that this is a highly recommended way to ease the trials and tribulations of overburdened, numerically inadequate, hospital and health personnel.

Community dentistry has a vital interest in auxiliary utilization and has stimulated much investigation in expanded duties. Cooperative exchanges and interrelationships should be explored and should result in even greater improvement in care.

Conclusion

The dentist's preoccupation with hosts of dental treatment problems has left little time for considering the perplexities of the dying or the dead patient's relatives. Community dentistry has now forced upon our consciousness the fact that perhaps the subject is one dentists need to stop avoiding if they are to fulfill completely their professional obligations to the public.

It is unfortunate that despite the long road the profession has traversed in scientific accomplishments, there still is a lingering reluctance to confront many of the problems of life and death. It is paradoxical that human beings should still speak about dying in dignity, and the dignity of death, and putting a person away in style, while the indignities perpetrated in life seem to be increasing, and interpersonal relationships remain brutal—even violent. It has been suggested that much of the contemporary mayhem may be the result of an unrealistic attitude towards dying and death.

Hopefully, in stimulating a greater understanding of death's problems and their ramifications, we might be able to assist in better understanding the difficulties of life, and thereby ease some of its burdens.

References

1. C. O. Dummett, "Community Dentistry, Also in the Modern Dental Curriculum," *Journal Southern California Dental Association,* Jan. 1969, pp. 23-31.

2. C. O. Dummett, "Providing Quality Care for the Nation," *Northwest Dentistry,* 49:294. Sept-Oct. 1970.

3. C. O. Dummett, "Understanding the Underprivileged Patient," *Journal American Dental Association,* 79:1363, Dec. 1969.

4. C. O. Dummett, "Community Dentistry's Contribution to Oral Care of Patients in Terminal Illness," (In Press).

Dental Needs of the Chronically Ill and Disabled Aged: As Seen by the Dental Hygienist

Georgia Hall [*]

Of the various health needs of the nation, none assumes more staggering proportions when measured by statistical evidence than dental disease. Of the various age groups none is more in need of attention, in terms of comprehensive and rehabilitative health care services, than the aged. There are more than fifteen million persons over the age of 65 in this country. At the present time, five per cent are in institutions (1). Oral health care of the chronically ill and disabled elderly is not given the attention it deserves. Proper dental care is an absolute necessity for the well-being of the chronically ill, disabled and institutionalized aged.

In many institutions today, medicine focuses sharply on the team approach to patient care. Newly admitted patients are considered at interdisciplinary conferences where staff members meet to discuss and plan their care. Quite often, however, one finds either that funds have not been allocated for dental services, or that all of the disciplines are not represented on the professional team. In many instances, the only professional person to examine the mouth of the elderly patient is the physician. A cursory examination, with notations on the medical chart concerning the degree of hydration of the oral tissues, will suffice. This may well be the only oral inspection the patient receives during his stay. If he is to be permanently institutionalized, this may be the last examination for the remainder of his life.

The general public, and even many members of the medical profession, are unaware of the need for periodic oral examinations by a dentist or hygienist for the elderly patient. Perhaps the dental profession is partly to blame. Oral health education is basically directed toward the young. Little is known of the need for periodic examinations of the denture-wearing patient.

The patient admitted to a nursing home may be recovering from a stroke, may have diabetes, and/or arteriosclerotic heart disease. He may be in need of total nursing care due to Parkinson's disease. He may suffer

[*] Formerly, Dental Hygienist, A. Holly Patterson Home for the Aged, Long Island, New York.

from generalized arteriosclerosis and chronic brain syndrome. He may present with diminished eyesight and sensory-neural hearing loss. Physical and mental disease are inextricably intertwined in aged patients (2). The appearance and state of health of the oral tissues mirror the patient's general state of health. Adequate nutrition and good hygiene are necessary for the maintenance of good oral health.

At the A. Holly Patterson Home for the Aged, comprehensive dental service is provided for all of that facility's 900 patients. The edentulous patient is very often surprised when asked to appear at the dental clinic for an examination. Even newly hired medical personnel will exclaim, "But he doesn't have any teeth," when they are asked to schedule such an examination. Approximately 60% of those admitted over a three-year period were edentulous, and a significant number of that group wore dentures. However, almost 100% of the denture-wearing group needed some form of dental treatment.

With age, biological changes are evident in all of the body tissues; the oral tissues are no exception. When full dentures have been worn for a significant length of time, the underlying alveolar bone undergoes resorption; the crests of the alveolar ridges lose height and the dentures become loose. This is particularly true for the mandibular jaw. Since the denture does not undergo any changes, the pressure of the ill-fitting prosthesis on the ridge causes injury to the tissue. In some individuals, this is manifested by redness and ulceration; in others, by hyperkeratinization of the tissue in the areas where the denture causes friction. The treatment should be either to reline the existing denture or to reconstruct a new one. If hyperkeratotic lesions are permitted to go untreated, they may develop into oral carcinoma. Seventy-five per cent of the hyperkeratotic lesions are found in persons 50 years of age and above; these are associated with chronic irritation (3). The anterior ridge of the maxilla is the site of irritational hyperplasia. This condition is also called Epulis fissuratum or compensatory hyperplasia. The tissue proliferates to compensate for the faulty adaptation of a denture flange. In treatment, the tissue must be excised and the denture corrected, if the patient's condition permits him to tolerate minor surgery.

The patient's medical history can be significant in terms of his oral health. The stroke patient who is no longer able to masticate bilaterally due to hemiplegia runs a greater risk of developing pathology on the afflicted side. The retention of food on that side predisposes the patient to carious lesions if natural teeth are present. The patient suffering from Parkinson's disease is more likely to retain food within the oral cavity due to dysphagia caused by rigidity of the laryngeal and pharyngeal muscles.

Special consideration must be given this patient when constructing replacement dentures.

Because diabetes mellitus in the older person is often associated with varying degrees of physical disability, he may require chronic maintenance care. Peripheral vascular disease, cerebral vascular disease or coronary thrombosis are often encountered (4). Although there is no proof, at present, as to the causal relationship of diabetes mellitus and increased gingival disease, the diabetic's tissues heal slowly and are less resistant to trauma and infection (5). Dental manipulation can precipitate infection of the periodontal structures. Preventive antibiotic therapy prior to and during dental treatment can be helpful.

The patient who presents with chronic brain syndrome, generalized arteriosclerosis or arteriosclerotic heart disease, may recall the details of events long past, but can forget that his teeth have not been brushed or his dentures removed and cleaned within the last few days. This patient must be supported continuously and assisted in maintaining his oral health.

Oral cancer comprises about 6% of all malignancies in the United States. Males are more susceptible and it is more common among the aged. Seventy-five per cent of the cases occur in persons over 50 years of age. Squamous cell carcinoma, which constitutes 90 to 95% of all mouth cancer, starts as a superficial ulcer or area of thickening (6). It is often associated with poor mouth hygiene and neglected teeth. Ill-fitting dentures have also been mentioned as being influential in the initiation of cancer of the mucous membranes, although little is known concerning the direct causation. Chronic irritation has been associated with oral cancer, but the etiological relationship has not been established. These findings must be kept in mind when treating the geriatric patient.

Various drugs frequently prescribed for the chronically ill, elderly patient, can have detrimental side effects. Penicillin, when taken over a protracted period of time, can cause monilial organisms present in the mouth to proliferate and result in oral moniliasis (thrush). The following will describe the findings of an oral examination of a newly admitted patient who had previously been receiving antibiotic therapy:

When Mrs. X, age 79, arrived at the dental clinic for her initial oral examination as a new resident, the nurse who accompanied her reminded the hygienist that Mrs. X had been feeling quite poorly for the past several days. The medical report designated the following:

1. Arteriosclerotic heart disease
2. Cardiomegaly
3. Chronic Cholycystitis with cholelithiasis
4. Osteoarthritis

Oral examination revealed the following:
1. Difficulty in opening the mouth
2. Edentulous—with full upper and lower vulcanite dentures in place
3. Buccal mucosa inflamed and appearing desquamatous
4. Removal of dentures obviously painful
5. Oral hygiene poor
6. All the tissues of the mouth and throat were found to be reddened with a sloughing off of a white, patch-like substance.

Since no dentist was on duty at the time, the hygienist immediately took the patient to the medical clinic where a physician was on duty. He suspected moniliasis and ordered a culture in appropriate solution for Candida albicans. In effect, that was it. She was advised to check the perineal area and a culture revealed the presence of the organisms there also. A three-week treatment with Nystatin effected a cure. The dentures were returned to the patient and she was given instruction as to their care. She is now able to eat well and to retain her food. She is in relatively good health.

Another side effect of continued drug therapy in the aged is xerostomia. The phenothiazine group of medications which include the commonly used tranquilizers have a desiccating effect on the oral mucous membrane. As a result of postmenopausal hormonal changes, many women suffer from xerostomia. This is further aggravated by mouth breathing. These patients must have the oral tissues frequently lubricated and fluids must be forced.

The majority of geriatric patients examined at the Patterson Home who were still in possession of their natural dentition had some degree of periodontal disease. This attacks the soft tissues around the teeth and the bone that supports them. The condition should be intercepted by frequent removal of calcareous deposits, curettage and polishing (prophylaxis). In addition, the patient should be maintained on an oral physiotherapy regime.

The teeth of the older person are not as vascular as those of the young. The pulp space is smaller; there is an increase in calcification and a loss of moisture. There is also an increase of fluorides in the dental enamel with advancing years. This may contribute to the reduction in dental caries in the teeth of the elderly (7). These factors tend to make the teeth more brittle. It is not uncommon to find a geriatric patient with several retained roots and crowns which have fractured and broken. These jagged remnants occasionally cannot be extracted due to the patient's physical condition or simply because he rejects extraction. His opinion must be honored. As long as there is no infection present and these teeth are functional, they may be ground and polished to prevent irritation of contiguous tissues. Not every person is to be considered a potential candidate for full-mouth extractions and the construction of dentures when he presents with this clinical picture.

It must be emphasized that each patient should be evaluated and treated as an individual. Therapeutic judgment exercised in treating a particular person may not be one and the same as clinical judgment. The patient must be considered clinically in his totality, even if the decision of the dentist seems to deny some of the basic principles of oral reconstruction and care.

So much is needed. Research should be conducted by dentists and hygienists with a sincere interest in the elderly in order to determine what biochemical changes occur in the oral structures of the aged. Dentists and hygienists should be made aware that the oral cavity consists of more than two rows of restorable teeth and that it is their responsibility to examine thoroughly all of the oral structures periodically. It is up to them to make their edentulous, denture-wearing patients aware of the need for periodic check-ups.

As a dental educator, it is up to the hygienist to disseminate information regarding oral health care of the elderly to senior citizen groups. All nursing homes should routinely provide dental services for their patients. Physicians should, in the absence of a dentist, take more time in examining the oral cavity and be more aware of normal as well as pathological conditions. Nursing staffs and their attendants must be made aware of the importance of daily mouth care for the total-care patient. It must be emphasized that this is incontestable as a part of total nursing care.

Perhaps the most important factor in the recognition of dentistry as a health service is that the mouth is an integral part of the body entity, and that an oral disease may either be the cause of or result in disorders of other parts of the body, especially in the geriatric patient.

References

1. J. L. Elmore, "Adaptation to Aging," *The Gerontologist, 10* (1):50, Part II, Spring, 1970.

2. B. A. Stotsky and J. R. Dominick, "The Physician's Role in the Nursing and Retirement Home," *The Gerontologist, 10*(1):38, Part II, Spring, 1970.

3. E. V. Zegarelli and A. H. Kutscher, *Diagnosis of Diseases of the Mouth and Jaws*, Philadelphia: Lea and Febiger, 1969.

4. J. L. Rudd and R. J. Margolin. *Maintenance Therapy for the Geriatric Patient*, Springfield: Charles C. Thomas, 1968.

5. E. M. Wilkins and P. A. McCullough, *Clinical Practice of the Dental Hygienist*, Philadelphia: Lea and Febiger, 1959.

6. L. R. Cahn and D. P. Slaughter, *Oral Cancer, a Monograph for the Dentist*, New York: American Cancer Society, Inc., 1962.

7. A. E. Elfenbaum, "Oral Care for the Elderly," *Proceedings of Seminars, 1965-69*, Duke University Council on Aging and Human Development, Duke University Medical Center, Durham, N.C., November, 1969.

Additional References

A. E. Elfenbaum, "April is Cancer Control Month," *Journal of the American Society for Geriatric Dentistry, 5 (2):*1, April, 1970.

Physician's Desk Reference, 24th Edition, Medical Economics, Inc., 1970.

Postoperative Nursing Care of Head-and-Neck Patients
*Alice Costello**

The goal and challenge in head and neck cancer nursing are to enable the patient to become independent, and all efforts are directed toward this end. A patient consents to surgery because of his desire to live and to obtain relief from pain. He fears not only the resultant cosmetic deformity and impairment of function but also the problem of acceptance by others. He does not need sympathy, but rather empathy and constructive help. The skilled, interested nurse with the ability to teach and help can simplify some of the problems involved. The patient should be encouraged to verbalize his needs and fears, but help should be given to guide him towards acceptance of full responsibility for his own care. It is *his* operation, and it is imperative that he learn to live with and adjust to it.

Many workers are involved in the patient's care. They include the surgeon, radiologist, dentist and/or prosthodontist, nurse, social worker and, if indicated, the chemotherapist and speech therapist. Rapport between the patient and caregivers is extremely important, as each has a contribution to make to the patient's care and recovery.

Following the surgical procedure the patient returns to the recovery room where nurses specially trained in the observation of symptoms, recording of data, and use of technical equipment are a valuable aid to him. The postoperative unit procedures consist of the following:

1. Semi Fowlers position to promote drainage and relieve edema.

2. Monitoring of blood pressure-pulse-respiration every 15 minutes.

3. A frequent check of the operative site for signs of hemorrhage.

4. Power suction at bedside with a Y tube set-up to which is attached a Yankauer suction tip for oral suction and a No. 16 whistle tip catheter for tracheal suction.

---

*Memorial Sloan Kettering Cancer Center, New York, New York.

5. Additional humidity to facilitate respiration and prevent formation of tracheal plugs.

6. Close attention to the cuffed tracheostomy tube. The balloon should be deflated upon leaving the operating room unless the patient is bleeding or receiving some form of positive pressure.

7. The inner part of tracheal tube should be removed at least every 1 to 2 hours, cleansed with soap and a nylon brush under running water and replaced.

8. Due to the danger of laryngeal spasm, which can result in fatal respiratory obstruction, only the doctor should remove the endotracheal tube when the patient has fully reacted.

9. Magic slate provided to enable the patient to communicate.

10. Checking Hemo-vac (closed system drainage) frequently to ascertain that drains are patent. Initially the drainage tubes are attached to a Gomco suction for 24 to 48 hours. Following this, the patient is placed on straight closed suction to remove the accumulation of serous and sanguinous fluid from beneath the skin flaps.

It is imperative that the head-and-neck patient be seen by the dentist pre-operatively, and it is one of the nurse's responsibilities to make sure that this is done. In all forms of intra-oral cancer, hygienic care of the oral cavity both before and during treatment is an important factor in successful care. Following surgery, the patient goes to the treatment room on the first postoperative day where power sprays (b.i.d.) of the oral cavity with dilute hydrogen peroxide followed by saline are initiated. The patient receiving pre- or postoperative radiation will have diluted Dobells solution substituted for H_2O_2. The milder Dobells solution is a combination of sodium borate, water, and glycerin and is less irritating to irradiated tissue.

The patient is provided with an oral irrigating set and is instructed to irrigate using a quart of warm water to which is added 1 teaspoon of salt and 1 teaspoon of sodium bicarbonate. Initially, he will irrigate 3 to 5 times daily. Following complete healing it may be necessary to irrigate only once a day or this may gradually be discontinued. As healing occurs, the patient is instructed to brush his teeth and, if his tongue is coated, he is told to procure a soft tooth brush and cleanse his tongue daily with tooth paste. Disposable soft foam rubber tooth brushes are excellent for this purpose. The importance of good oral hygiene in helping to reduce edema, alleviate pain and discomfort, and prevent or resolve infection cannot be overemphasized. For the patient with a local infection in the floor of the mouth or buccal gutter, zinc peroxide packs have proved extremely efficacious. This powder has been activated and is mixed with water to form a smooth paste. Depending upon the area to be treated a 4x4, 2x2, or 1 inch gauze packing is impregnated and placed over the area of infection. The packing is then changed every 2 hours. For the patient with a dry crusting mouth, following extensive radiation therapy, glycerine and lemon swabs, which the patient sucks like a lollipop, have been found to be helpful. It is also suggested that the patient with this condition suck lemon or peppermint drops.

Following surgery and the patient's temporary inability to swallow, a No. 18 French 2-holed feeding tube is passed. The first tube passed is by the doctor and subsequent tubes by the nurse. Eventually, the patient is taught to pass his own feeding tube by inserting it straight along the floor of the nasal cavity, directing it horizontally backwards until it reaches the oral cavity and turns downward. At this point, a "plop" will be experienced and the patient then makes the motion of swallowing and assists the passage of the tube into the esophagus. In order to secure the tube properly, so that it will not pass into the stomach, a Martin Pitou nasal phlange is used which is secured by means of a rubber band and paper tape to the nose or cheek. In order to insure proper positioning, the feeding tube is always checked. While hospitalized, the patient is taught to feed himself using a plastic funnel with a rubber tube. The funnel is held at eye level to prevent flatus resulting from a too rapid passage of the food into the stomach. In the hospital, a funnel stand is used; however, it is suggested that upon discharge, the patient purchase an ordinary tooth brush and glass holder which can be attached to a wall at the proper height and is ideal for holding the funnel.

Approximately 25% of oral cancer patients require some form of prosthetic appliance. The best example of the functional prosthesis is the intra-oral obturator. Since wound contracture following a partial or radical maxillectomy is rapid in the early stages, both the hospital and clinic nurse should be cognizant of this hazard and caution the patient against removing the appliance for a prolonged period. The prosthesis should be worn even at night and removed only in order to cleanse it. The nurse instructs the patient that the obturator's function is to enable him to eat, speak and swallow. It prevents food passing from the oral into the nasal cavity, thus helping to avoid painful infection and making the postoperative course more comfortable.

For the patient with a radical maxillectomy and/or orbital exenteration, the insertion of a fluffed 4x4 gauze moistened with mineral oil into the defect has been found to be an effective method of helping to keep the area clean and free of crusts. The nurse should also be alert to a pyocyanosis or "Green Bug" infection which is a particular complication of skin grafts of the maxillary defect. Sprays of 1% acetic acid followed by acid packs should be started at the first sign of this infection. Tracheitis sicca is a particular complication of laryngectomized and tracheostomy patients. It is caused by cold dry air and results in an accumulation of dried mucous plugs, crusts and bleeding. The patient is instructed to turn the heat off in the bedroom at night, use a steam vaporizer, and always wear a moistened gauze bib over the stoma. Should sicca develop, a 5% sodium bicarbonate solution is sprayed into the stoma to help dissolve the crusts; mucomist may be ordered by the physician; and the patient is placed on intensive steam inhalation therapy. In severe sicca, it is sometimes necessary to bronchoscope the patient and remove the plugs manually.

Due to the nerve and muscle resections necessitated by the radical neck procedure, the patient develops a shoulder drop and forward curvature which may result in a frozen shoulder if this is not corrected promptly. In order to help prevent this, the patient is started on a series of exercises as soon as the neck flaps are adhered. Instructions should be given on a one-to-one basis, and, in demonstrating the exercise, the importance of relaxation emphasized. The patient repeats the demonstration and any errors are corrected. On subsequent visits, the patient's progress is observed and any necessary follow-up teaching is done.

The greatest service nurses can render the head-and-neck patient is to teach him to be self-sufficient regarding his own care. This will give him a feeling of self-confidence, help him accept the results of his surgery more readily and facilitate his return to society. This is both the goal and the challenge in cancer nursing. Naturally, it is not accomplished in one lesson; it requires constant reiteration of principles, supervision of the procedures to be performed, endless patience and encouragement. Patients fear not only the surgery with the resulting cosmetic deformity and impairment of function, but their acceptance by others. Therefore, the nurse's ability to teach, guide and help to simplify their problems is an invaluable asset.

Rapport with the family members is also essential. They too need help in accepting and adjusting to the surgery which has been performed. The nurse instructs them on how to assist the patient with the various procedures he will need to perform at home. They should be given a sense of participation in the patient's treatment and rehabilitation and assured of the nurse's interest. Both the patient and his family should be given a sense of security by being urged to maintain contact with the hospital staff concerning any problems that might arise. Simultaneously, the normal inclination of many family members towards overprotectiveness must be discouraged.

The care of the terminal patient is psychologically traumatic to *everyone* involved. The patient facing death wants to live and needs more than professional competence. He needs insight, compassion and, above all, an assurance of the nurse's interest in him as an individual person. The nurse's obligation is to help him face death, when this comes to pass, in peace and with dignity.

Nursing Care and Interpersonal Relationships

Madelaine A. Bader [*]

The professional nurse renders a unique role as she fulfills her responsibility for service to dying patients, their families and the nursing staff. It is the physician who makes determinations in the areas of diagnosis, prognosis or prescribing treatments for disease. The nurse, however, is the authority for nursing care. Nursing care is developed by nurses and nursing service assumes primary responsibility for it. Nurses have the particular obligation and commitment to determine, plan, implement, supervise, evaluate and modify nursing care. The professional nurse, unlike any other health worker, devotes herself to the continuous care of the patient in order to meet his needs.

A helpful definition in defining the function of a professional nurse is Henderson's concept of nursing:

> The unique function of the nurse is to assist the individual, sick or well, in the performance of those activities contributing to health or its recovery (or to a peaceful death) that he would perform unaided if he had the necessary strength, will or knowledge. And to do this in such a way as to help him gain independence as rapidly as possible (1).

It is the professional nurse who maintains a constancy and coordination of services. Doctors, clergy, social workers and others come and go. Only the nurse continues those services affecting human life around the clock. Possessing and using a disciplined intellectual approach in combination with a therapeutic use of self, she is also the person most likely to become immediately involved with the patient's problems (2).

The use of the disciplined intellectual approach with patients means that the professional nurse is able to draw upon and use concepts and principles from the natural, physical, biological, behavioral, nursing and medical sciences. Moreover, by means of her disciplined intellectual approach, she is able to put this knowledge into practice with

---

[*]Lieutenant Colonel, Army Nurse Corps, Chief, Clinical Nursing Section, Psychiatry and Neurology, Walter Reed Army Medical Center, Washington, D.C.

understanding. A therapeutic framework for nursing intervention, based on the needs of the patient, is used to plan, implement and evaluate nursing care.

To be successful, a disciplined intellectual approach for patient care must be employed in combination with therapeutic use of self. The former focuses largely on theory, while therapeutic use of self concerns the very process of nursing, that is, what is happening between the nurse and the patient. Therapeutic use of self can be defined as the ability to use one's personality and knowledge consciously in order to effect a change in the patient's behavior. This change is considered therapeutic when it lessens the dying patient's sense of isolation, despair and hopelessness.

The nurse needs to recognize that the fear of dying operates within herself as well as within the patient. Only when the nurse becomes aware of some of the fears that dying and death hold for her, can she begin to comprehend and "feel" what a life-threatening illness may mean to her patient. It is perhaps only then that she can begin the process of asking herself what she can do *for* and *with* the dying person, based on his needs, to help him live his remaining life in a way most meaningful to him: to consider ways she might assist him to "become"; to resolve his unfinished business; and to die in peace and with dignity.

The insights and understandings she develops about herself can be consciously and therapeutically used in the ways she relates to the dying person. In actual practice, both of the abilities—a disciplined intellectual approach and therapeutic use of self—are operant and one influences the other as the professional nurse works with the person who has a life-threatening illness.

Techniques are often used by the nurse and nursing personnel to facilitate relationships. Techniques in themselves, however, are not enough. When the meaning behind a patient's behavior is evaluated in terms of what it *means* to *him*, the techniques can be employed therapeutically. The nurse then is in the position to assist the patient towards accomplishment of his purpose in a healthier manner through the use of a selected technique.

The following clinical example will illustrate how the professional nurse identifies patient needs, implements nursing care measures and evaluates effectiveness of care in order to assist the patient to regain equilibrium and learn a new way of coping with his symptoms and feelings. It also serves to illustrate how continuous assessment of the patient's behavior helps the nurse to plan her approach, based on theory, so his needs can be met. Physical, interpersonal, and behavioral cues given by the patient determine when the nurse can intervene and offer a new learning experience to the patient.

> Hugh H., a twenty-three-year-old married man and father, had been admitted to the hospital that morning. His first admission, several months ago, had been for treatment of Hodgkin's disease. Since discharge he had been followed on an outpatient basis. The present admission was precipitated by gastro-intestinal distress accompanied by intermittent vomiting, diarrhea, fever, and resultant dehydration. When the nurse walked in the large ward, Hugh was lying on his back in bed. His face reflected anguish and he kept nervously biting his lower lip as though to keep from calling out. Evidence that he was fearful of losing control was indicated by the following kinds of statements: "I can't stand this any longer—this pain in my chest. God! When are they going to give me something that will kill the pain? I feel like I'm being pulled in all different directions." The nurse recognized the patient's need for structure and began to reduce the patient's anxiety to a manageable level by identifying the need through verbal recognition of the patient's felt concern for controls. She told the patient that she and the nursing staff were here to assist him in maintaining control. For this particular patient, medication was the initial technique used, accompanied by emotional support, to provide control and strengthen defenses. One hour later, as the nurse evaluated the effectiveness of planned care, she noted that the patient appeared troubled. Hugh's face appeared tense, his jaw muscles twitched, stretching the skin over his cheekbones. His curt "yes" to her query about the effectiveness of the pain medication seemed incongruous with his expression. She knew Hugh had not anticipated this admission. (The doctors had planned on having Hugh return to the hospital on an inpatient basis for treatment with another new experimental drug and viewed this admission, once he was over his gastric distress, as an opportunity to institute the new protocol. The doctors told him about the new plan of treatment on rounds.) The nurse attempted to "walk through" the past twenty-four hours as though she were the patient. She then expressed these feelings to Hugh, "I was just imagining how I might feel had I been in your place returning to the hospital this morning. It would have kicked off a whole host of fantasies for me. Did it kick any off for you?" Hugh glanced quickly at the nurse, touched her arm and sighed a long "Yes, I thought, 'Oh Boy, here we go again, Hugh baby. The tumor's growing back in the chest. It's getting larter." (His hands were alternately clutching the bedclothes, touching the nurse's arm, and moving rapidly over his chest.) "The doctors stopped and told me the X-rays revealed nothing has changed. I'd like to believe them, but why do I still have pain? They said while I'm here they are going to try a new drug on me. I had planned on going home in a couple of days. Now I can't."

He continued to talk for the next fifteen minutes. He began to speak less rapidly, body gestures were less exaggerated, and posture appeared more relaxed. Hugh continued, "I guess maybe the medicine is helping now. Hey! It's gone! My chest pain is gone!" (The nurse had been repeatedly assessing Hugh's level of anxiety and now evaluated it to be mild. The nurse used this assessment to assist the patient in learning something different about himself.) She asked Hugh, "Is the medicine the only reason you feel better inside?" Hugh replied, "I think so. What else could it be? Well, maybe the pain was due to the tension of coming back to the hospital and thinking the throwing up and diarrhea was because the tumor was growing again. (Hesitated.) Well, it might also be because I talked about how I felt. I never do that, you know. You seemed interested in understanding me and you listened. I guess talking about how I felt did help. I don't feel so angry inside." A few minutes later, the patient fell asleep.

The verbalization of unexpressed emotion had the value of some relief of emotional tension. and the patient began to feel understood and accepted by another person. Moreover, the nurse, by determining the patient's need for control and validating her observation, helped the patient to link events and feelings with reactions and symptoms—a linkage which the patient had not previously recognized on his own. The increase in the patient's understanding and partial insight may lead to an increase in perspective and objectivity, as well as to a lessening of anxiety and some undercutting of future automatic responses. The nurse, through supportive therapy, used those interpersonal techniques which made the patient feel more secure, reassured, accepted, encouraged, protected, safe, less anxious and less alone.

Working with Others

Studies of social structure demonstrate that staff interaction influences patient care. As leader of the nursing team, the professional nurse is in a position to assist other members in the therapeutic use of self so that they, too, can make a contribution to the care of the dying person. With her academic background and experience in human behavior, she is able to advise and participate with fellow staff members in relation to the emotional, interpersonal and physiological factors involved in various kinds of nursing problems. The professional nurse explores her behavior toward and emotional responses to dying patients, including the negative as well as positive ones, and shares these feelings with her nursing staff. As a result, the nursing staff members tend to feel more secure in revealing their own negative and positive feelings and reactions about dying patients.

The team members, who are dependent upon one another for effective results, must work harmoniously together. This requires a sharing of responsibilities and of strengths, a spirit of give-and-take, and a sense of mutual respect. The professional nurse is responsible for promoting harmonious relationships among members of the nursing team and assisting them in exploring the anxieties which may arise in coping with one another. For instance, if interpersonal conflict arises among staff members, the nurse provides leadership to examine and assess what is going on in the situation that caused the conflict, and to help them in identifying the source of the conflict so that it may be resolved.

Furthermore, the nurse must be sensitive to all staff interactions, the factors which promote harmony as well as those which tend to separate members. The nurse needs to realize that when problems arise with the staff members, their sense of security is threatened. The cohesiveness of the nursing staff is jeopardized and discouragement, disappointment and anger result. Unless the nurse recognizes the problem and assists staff members to recognize and deal with their feelings, rather than avoid them, the quality of patient care will suffer. Indeed, the dying patient may well become the recipient of the staff's anxiety.

Through staff conferences staff members can be afforded an opportunity to clarify their interactions and feelings. These conferences can be used as opportunities for staff to discuss feelings and the impact upon relationships, work out differences, and arrive at satisfactory solutions which hopefully will aid staff members in developing greater objectivity in practice. When the energy of the staff is tied up defending its sense of security and worth, the members are less able to extend themselves to the concerns of dying patients. Only as members of the nursing team are helped to learn and understand their own anxieties and fears of death can they assist dying patients with theirs.

The professional nurse can influence the quality of care that dying patients receive by presenting herself as a role model to staff and patients. By her manner of address and reference to dying patients, a feeling of maintaining individual dignity is adopted by other personnel.

Additionally, the professional nurse collaborates, validates and shares patient data with the physician and other health disciplines. Her attitude that, "We are working together, I have this to give, I need this from you," is central to promoting a better understanding by others of the importance of dealing with the fear of death, the threat of death and its effect upon the dying patient.

It is through these kinds of interactions among staff members that the dying patient can begin to experience an atmosphere of acceptance, trust and security. Opportunities are provided to view his behavior more objectively because the staff promotes the kinds of experiences that lessen his need for continuing his present pattern of behavior, be it withdrawal, denial, anger, depression or a blend of all of these. These experiences permit the dying patient to acquire a more realistic understanding of himself, his environment and his relationships with others, and enable him to begin expressing his fears and concerns, including the possibility of death.

It should not be forgotten that patients with life-threatening llnesses are also members of a family. What affects dying patients affects family structure and a resultant temporary disequilibrium among family members is often observed. One should no more neglect considering the kind of help families need in mastering this situation than one would neglect to consider the kinds of help patients need which may determine the direction and course of their care.

Families perceive the nurse as the one professional person who is always in attendance. Because nurses are frequently perceived by the family members as people who give comfort and care to their loved one, nurses are in a favorable position to maximize their influence in assisting families to cope more effectively with life-threatening illnesses.

There are certain opportunities that may occur with the family during the first few hours or days of the loved one's admission that may not occur later in his hospitalization. These opportunities revealed by interactions, if recognized by the nurse, will help her form a base for establishing a meaningful relationship with the family. This relationship can be maintained and strengthened throughout the patient's hospitalization, with the nurse serving as helper, advisor and confidant to the family members when they begin to deal with the various aspects of their loved one's illness and possible death. Several clinical examples illustrate how needs can be manifested through these kinds of opportunities and how nurses meet these needs.

Feelings may be particularly pronounced in family members during this initial time period. They may be concerned over their lack of firsthand knowledge about the hospital's physical plant, which heightens their feeling of insecurity. They worry about the condition of their loved one and the kinds of care he might receive. One wife, whose husband had suddenly became comatose at home, expressed her feelings in this fashion:

> We landed at Andrews Air Force Base and they immediately whisked my husband off the flight line, put him in an ambulance and took him to Walter Reed General Hospital. I waited in the airplane until someone told me to go into the terminal. Someone, I don't really know who, told me to stay right there and I did. Soon a soldier came by and directed me to the Army bus that was leaving for Walter Reed. When I arrived at Walter Reed they told me my husband was on Ward X. I asked for directions and someone told me how to get to the ward. The nurse on the ward met me as I entered and told me the doctors were with my husband and soon I'd be able to see him. She hugged me and told me she hoped everything would be all right. When she did that, I sort of knew he'd have a chance. She arranged a room for me at the Guest House. I hadn't even thought of where I might stay. I was just worried about Pa and how he was doing.

Although this woman did not enlarge upon her statement, the implication might well be, "It's a good feeling to know that someone is concerned about my husband and me. The kind of caring for what happens to Pa made all the difference in the world—made me feel like he's in good hands."

A husband expressed his feeling of dismay and isolation when he said, "I didn't know if I would be able to see my wife more than the five minutes every hour indicated on the sign outside of the intensive care unit. A nurse saw me pacing outside, spent some time with me telling me about my wife's care and then explained that the five minute visit limitation was flexible depending on each patient's need. What a relief to know I could probably see her more frequently."

Other opportunities available to nurses and nursing personnel during the first few hours or days the family of a patient with a life-threatening illness is on a unit involved dealing with similar kinds of incidents. Once needs are determined for a particular family, a vast reservoir of helping people can be called upon to give assistance. For some families, the doctor may be the crucial person; for others it might be the chaplain; for yet others the Red Cross worker or the social worker would be the essential person to contact. When nurses recognize the threats in the environment that increase stress to family members, measures can be taken to abort possible threats to the family's security, self-esteem, judgment, need for warmth and affection, and identity as people.

Project CAM (Crisis Awareness and Management) at Walter Reed Army Medical Center makes a special contribution in expediting the expansion of awareness among hospital workers as they deal with death and dying. Project CAM began in late September, 1970, through the combined efforts of a psychiatric nurse and a social worker, as a framework for eventual involvement of an interdisciplinary crisis team to assist people who care for the dying patient and his family.

The purpose of the crisis team was twofold: 1) to conduct teaching seminars with personnel who deal with crises situations; and 2) to send one or more members of the team to wards *requesting* guidance concerning the management of crises in either staff, patient or his family.

The teaching seminars were designed to promote a sharing of attitudes, approaches and insights among the participants responsible for the care of the dying person and his family. It was hoped that such seminars would create an atmosphere in which staff members could begin to deal with their feelings about death. Guideliness and approaches would be discussed so personnel would become more effective in dealing with terminally ill patients. It was hoped that increased sensitivity and perceptiveness among personnel would develop to meet the needs of the terminally ill patient and his family, and the need both would have for increased psychological support at that time; and that an awareness and sensitivity would develop among staff members regarding the necessity for them also to have a period of mourning and grieving when a patient dies.

While we realize that death may well be the most difficult issue for all health team members to handle, death is merely one of the many crises involving loss. We, therefore, work with the health team to focus initially on death, our rationale being that having assisted them to work through some of their feelings regarding this most critical manifestation of loss, they may then find it easier to deal effectively with other lesser manifestations of loss—be it financial, body part, organ, role or relationship.

Each weekly seminar, similar to those developed and described by Dr. Kubler-Ross (3) essentially followed this format:

The first hour: Viewing via closed circuit TV a live video interview conducted by the psychiatric nurse and the social worker with a terminally ill patient and/or his family.

The second hour: After the patient and the family have left, the nurse and social worker join the participants to share "gut level" reactions and feelings about the interview and invite the participants to do likewise.

The discussions include crisis theory, management, patient and family needs, approaches and guidelines one might use, and discussion of feelings about one's own death. Heavy emphasis is given to Dr. Kubler-Ross' work concerning theory and behavioral manifestations of loss. A selected bibliography with handouts is given participants.

Reactions from participants (included were a doctor, social workers, psychologists, nurses, a speech therapist, and chaplains) were most favorable. Requests for assistance and guidance began coming from nurses on wards who had heard about Project CAM. At first only doctors known to the participants called. As the project has continued, other doctors, nursing supervisors and faculty members from the School of Nursing have joined the program.

When referrals come from a ward, the patient or the family is seldom seen. Instead, work is done with the staff members on that ward. Our expectations are that staff members will be able to work with the patient and his family. If we worked directly with the patient or his family, we might deprive the staff of a potentially growth-producing situation. Our process of intervention follows: we gather as many of the staff as possible and go to an empty room or lounge area. First, clarification of the ward composition is sought—veterans, beginners, students or others. Inquiries are made about staff workload. The details of the patient's illness and what staff members may know about this family are discussed. Staff members are then asked if they can identify the major feelings just expressed. Identifying feelings at this point results in further clarification, catharsis, and movement towards whatever elements may indirectly be causing upset in staff members.

Frequent comments are, "I am angry, anxious or depressed," and subsequently, "A death will mean we've failed again, maybe we just didn't do all we could for him." Rarely do we hear, "I am angry or anxious because the patient makes me aware of my own mortality." However, we seek to promote and develop insight in this area. When we can bring to awareness what has indirectly caused the upset—fear of one's death, anger, or depression stemming from the inability to sustain life—it is then quite natural to promote insight among staff members concerning the reasons for the patient's behavior and that of his family.

It may be necessary to allow staff members to air angry feelings before problem solving can begin. When staff members ask, "OK, what do we do now?", the session becomes a learning experience for all. We might offer suggestions or guidelines to staff which we feel may be useful. However, it is up to the staff to decide whether the suggestions can be utilized at that time. Staff members are encouraged to go as far as their knowledge and experience will take them. This is done to promote group interaction and cohesiveness so that in future crisis situations group strengths again might be used effectively (4).

The following vignette serves to illustrate the kind of contribution Project CAM has been making to wards in terms of facilitating expansion of awareness among health workers in dealing with dying patients:

> It was at the beginning of the fifth session of the seminar series that I was confronted by one of the participants, a head nurse, who said, "I have the perfect situation for you." She described briefly a terminally ill patient who was causing her and her staff concern. We spoke briefly for I was on my way to meet the patient we were to interview. I left thinking we must make time the second hour for that head nurse to share the situation with her fellow participants. Fortunately, as it happened later, the patient we were to interview could not come due to last minute tests that had been ordered. (When situations like these occur, we use a back-up video tape of a previous interview which has been selected for its relevance at that point in the series.) I shared with the social worker what the head nurse had mentioned. We decided to join the group and use the situation the head nurse had briefly sketched to me, rather than the video tape. The discussion that followed was lively and all members became actively involved. The head nurse, when the discussion concluded, asked for guidance and support so she could work with her staff and together they could plan care for this patient. Arrangements were made to visit the ward the following day.

> When I arrived, Mrs. S. called her staff together for a meeting in the lounge. That morning the meeting was attended by the head nurse, staff nurse, and three non-professional personnel. The meeting lasted slightly over an hour. The first forty minutes were spent in describing the patient's behavior and treatment. The patient was a woman in her forties with metastatic cancer. Although she had been treated with radiation and chemotherapy, her response to treatment was negligible. She had been confined to a wheelchair for several weeks. It was the feeling of the health team and her doctor that she had only a "short time" to live. The husband was perceived by staff as an angry man who forever was finding fault with the care and treatment his wife received. The wife was described as a lady who had episodes of confusion. She often appeared angry with staff members. Staff members told about a remark she made when one of them entered her room to inquire how she felt. She responded, "You're just coming in here to check and see if I'm still living." Staff members felt

they had tried all approaches and nothing worked. They were afraid that her husband might report them to higher authorities and wanted me to intervene. I shared with them my feelings that they would be able to work with this woman and her husband and suggested we talk more about feelings.

The nursing team began to relate personal losses they had experienced and how they reacted to them. Toward the end of the hour, I asked them if the patient had ever talked about dying. One practical nurse responded, "Yes, but when she asked me if she was going to die, her husband spoke right up and told her she wasn't going to die. I didn't have a chance to say anything." We did a short role-playing episode of how she might have responded if the husband had not been present. This seemed to touch a response in several staff members. We speculated on ways we might be able to help the husband communicate with his wife so they could begin to share the remaining time together in a way most meaningful to them. At this point, the head nurse said, "I've never in the past given him a straightforward answer when he asked me if his wife would ever be well. I always hedged. I feel now he really wanted to know. Perhaps the next time I'll be able to answer him."

The session ended with several suggestions: 1) staff members might visit with Mrs. X. at times other than when they had to do something for her. This might hold great meaning for her in terms of perceiving staff as persons who care what happens to her, and 2) rather than waiting for the husband to come out of his wife's room and ask staff what they had done for her, to attempt to meet him before he visited her, and give him a report of what had transpired since his last visit. I left the ward with an invitation from staff to return the following week at the same time.

When I arrived on the ward the following week, the head nurse, Mrs. S, met me and said, "Mr. X. asked yesterday morning if his wife was any better. This time I was able to tell him that her condition remained the same. He seemed satisfied with my answer and went to visit his wife. A short time later he came out and told me he was on his way downtown to purchase a wig that would cover the bald spot his wife had due to the treatments. This is the first time Mr. X. has ever left the ward during daytime hours. Maybe the fact that we've been informing him the past week about his wife's care before he had to ask increased his security and trust in the staff."

The second session consisted of exploring both positive and negative feelings evoked when one works with patients who are dying. At this meeting, the composition of the group consisted of two professional nurses, five non-professional nursing assistants and two nursing students. Staff members were reluctant to share "gut level" feelings until I shared my own feeling of disgust over the smell that emanated from a patient with a colostomy who had died on their ward several months ago. With this, staff members began sharing their negative feelings—something they said they never had done before. They seemed surprised to discover they had negative feelings. Toward the end of the session, we talked about Mrs. X. and what she might be feeling at this stage in her illness. Staff members talked about her wish to go to her retirement home in Florida—a home she had never seen. One licensed practical nurse remarked thoughtfully, "You know, she just might get to Florida after all. I capitalized on her statement and reinforced it by saying, "If you think she might get to Florida, and if you and you and you think she might get there, then by God she just might, for she will be picking up the hope you have for her—and who are we to say she won't make it and take away that hope?" Nursing personnel again invited me back for another meeting the following week.

When I arrived on the ward, I was met by one of the nursing assistants who rather pointedly commented, "We've been waiting for you. You're one minute late" I was escorted to the lounge flanked by nurses and nursing assistants—a most unusual happening. They sat down and looked at me most expectantly. I asked the question they all seemed to be waiting for, "How is Mrs. X?" The entire nursing staff chimed, "Would you believe she has a wig, is walking, and the doctor is going to discharge her this weekend?" Each member's face looked as though she had experienced Christmas and New Year's simultaneously and couldn't wait to share with me the good news. "And you know how we thought she was confused—she wasn't at all. That man she sometimes talked about was our own custodian. We never knew Mr. B's name. She said he was the only one that would ever just chat with her, that is, until a week or so ago." I shared my joy and delight with them and said, "Well what do you suppose made the difference? Because if you can figure out what made the difference with Mrs. X. when a similar kind of situation occurs, you'll be able to utilize what you've learned and apply it to someone else." Twenty minutes were spent as staff members delineated factors that may have made the difference. Although many factors were mentioned, the one fact which kept recurring was the change in the attitude of all staff members—an attitude change from one of despair and giving up to an attitude of hope for Mrs. X. Result: Mrs. X. is going home. She still has the disease, but the hope she has experienced from staff was the tree of life for her, and that completed her universe. Staff members had actually created an atmosphere where hope could flourish.

With hope, all things are possible—even going home.

References

1. V. Henderson, *The Nature of Nursing*, New York: The Macmillan Company, 1966, p. 15.
2. J. Travelbee, *Interpersonal Aspects of Nursing*, Philadelphia: F. A. Davis Company, 1966, p. 14.
3. E. Kubler-Ross, *Death and Dying*, New York; The Macmillan Company, 1969.
4. M. A. Bader and R. P. Flaherty, "Project CAM (Crisis Awareness and Management) Crisis team begins at Walter Reed Army Medical Center," Unpublished paper, 1971.

Oral Care of the Dying Patient: A Social Worker's Point of View

Evelyn F. Cooper*

In today's world no aspect of human experience escapes scrutiny. Birth, sex, aging and death, processes which in the past have been regarded as being either of a highly professional or highly personal nature, are now in the public domain. The result is a growing inter-relationship between professional practice and consumer demands, out of which has arisen increasing recognition of the need for a better human condition.

Oral care of the dying patient may be considered under two categories. First, there is the group of patients whose primary disease involves the oral cavity, such as patients with carcinoma of the tongue or floor of the mouth. The need for oral hygiene as well as rehabilitative measures is obvious in these patients and considerable attention is given them by the professional personnel involved. The second class of oral care needs are those of terminally ill patients whose major disease lies elsewhere than in the mouth. Minor and major problems of routine dental care and oral hygiene are of immeasurable significance to the sense of physical and emotional well-being of each of these patients. However, there seems to be a widespread, often tacit, feeling of futility about planning for dental care of patients with limited life expectancy—it appears to be regarded as an investment not justified by the returns. Perhaps, too, the pedestrian quality of this service deprives it of any sense of drama or professional challenge so that such care more easily becomes a potential area of neglect. Yet the concept of comprehensiveness of care surely implies no difference in its application to those who will not recover from their illness than it does for those who will. Failure to provide comprehensive care is tantamount to failure to meet standards established by professionals themselves.

For purposes of this discussion, the "dying" patient is the patient with an irreversible illness, an illness that is actively progressing and will inevitably cause the patient's death. Because of the variety of illnesses which may be terminal, it is obvious that time considerations will vary from case to case. Heart disease, neurological disease and cancer are illnesses of such gravity and critical concern to those treating the patient

---

* Director, Social Service Department, Memorial Hospital for Cancer and Allied Diseases, New York, New York.

that preoccupation with the treatment of the primary condition often overshadows those problems of seemingly secondary importance in the well-being of the patient. This need not be an inevitable pitfall. We well know that advances in the methods of treatment of patients with irreversible illnesses are continually prolonging patients' survival; the quality of this survival should not be overlooked. Health professionals in particular have a responsibility for implementing measures which will enable the patient to use all of his faculties, optimally and productively, for as long as possible. Attitudes of professionals are readily communicated to the patient and it will bolster him to feel our conviction that he is still in the mainstream of living. Serious illness need not deprive one of the pleasures of ties with family, of assuming responsibility, and of making decisions.

Oral care and proper dentition can be factors in the patient's physical comfort as well as aids in his nutrition and contributing factors to his sense of personal dignity. Presumably, there is no disagreement that like good skin care for the chronically ill, good mouth care is essential. However, skin breakdown in the chronically ill can be detected readily by professional personnel or by family members; failures of oral hygiene tend to be less obvious. Hence the interest in oral care must be built into the system of generalized patient care. Proper mouth care may well have much to do with the personal standards and life-long habits of an individual. If the patient has been exposed to good standards of personal and oral hygiene from an early age, it is quite likely that with the functional ability to do so, he will make an effort to continue what he has deemed necessary, or if he becomes dependent on others, he will seek assistance. However, if socioeconomic and/or psychological conditions have created a lack of impetus for such care, then the patient is not likely to expect it or ask for it.

Society must place a new value on the adequate dental care of the general population. Those social workers who deal with the medically indigent and the indigent know only too well the problems associated with obtaining dental services. Dental care as a criterion of health is not considered to be essential. We have ample evidence of this in the fact that provision by public agencies for dental care is only for the most acute conditions, dental services in hospitals exist for the "emergency situations" of patients who are under treatment in the institution for other reasons, and dental care is not usually included in health insurance policies. The fact is that many people regard dental care as something of a luxury; an impression that is borne out by the fact that dental practice is by and large a private office practice "enjoyed" by the middle and upper classes.

The social worker's responsibility in the care of the dying patient is carried out in collaboration with the appropriate medical, nursing and other personnel who are also involved in the patient's care. The social worker's focus is on the patient as an individual and as a member of a family. The chronically ill patient is caught in a maze of physical weakness, painful therapeutic procedures, changed physical appearance, and prolonged dependency. He is easy prey to feelings of being burdensome to his family and society and to feeling isolated and worthless. By learning from the patient himself what changes his illness has created for both him and his family, the social worker attempts to buttress the patient's links with the world around him and reinforce his self-esteem. What might be understood in the course of this process is what oral neglect means to a patient.

We are all subtly influenced by our own values (or prejudices) and these are often unintentionally reflected in the priorities we manifest in the care of patients. For example, are we assuming that since routine mouth care can be self-administered, it is being provided? Is it assumed that the patient will always ask for what he wants and needs? On a busy hospital floor which is short of staff, might a patient be labelled a "nag" if he complained about his mouth being dry or not being able to eat properly? Might he not be dubbed "orally-centered" and ignored? Has any hospital not had the experience of a patient who was relieved of his dentures before a specific procedure—"We'll wrap them in Kleenex and put them away so they won't get lost,"—and he never sees them again? Are the patient's comments about his mouth reported in his medical chart so that when his doctor makes rounds he will become aware of the problem? As noted above, advancing disease can cover a long period of time and allow for varying degrees of functioning. Whether a patient is at home, in a hospital, or in a nursing home facility, the standard of his care should certainly convey that the professionals treating him have an active concern that he obtain the benefit of all known therapies, that efforts in his behalf will not be relinquished, and that attention will be given to his physical, emotional, and environmental comfort. Thus, a healthy self-interest can be maintained in the patient and we will find that he is ready to participate in self-care rather than to slip into early dependency.

It is not only the patient who is in need of these assurances but the family as well. During the course of the patient's illness, the family very likely has made many adjustments—not only to the changes the illness has created for the patient, but changes in the pattern of family life. Catastrophic illness brings changes in the responsibilities of family members, changes in the physical arrangements of a household, economic problems, emotional strains. At times, family members are torn with guilt; at other times, they are enraged over their burdens. One of the small sources of satisfaction they may have is the conviction that they are doing everything to give the patient the best possible care.

Social workers are well aware that the social deprivation and the isolation that is a concomitant of terminal illness can cause as much debilitation in the patient as the disease process itself. Communication with the patient in order to create a climate of individualized care is the *sine qua non* for avoiding these damaging experiences. In communication there is sharing of thoughts, relieving feelings, maintaining one's identity, satisfying one's wants. These are some of the by-products of good oral care, for when practice within an institution provides for multidisciplinary patient care, there is greater likelihood that the whole spectrum of patient needs will receive visibility; with this mechanism the psychosocial observations of all of the health professionals can be pooled and assessed in terms of patient needs.

The patient with head-and-neck disease will, of course, most likely have meticulous care for his oral problems. While these patients represent only a small segment of the total patient (terminal) population, it is instructive to examine how crucial the application of a team concept can be with irreversible illness.

> A 28-year-old man first sought help from a dentist when his symptoms appeared; a differential diagnosis by the dentist brought him proper care for his cancer. After he underwent surgery for an osteogenic sarcoma of the left maxillary antrum, his speech was severely impaired. This young man was a playwright and not to be able to speak was an overwhelming frustration. Until it was possible for him to be fitted with a maxillary prosthesis, the social worker recognized with him that for an individual with his "articulate nature" his handicap in speech was an almost unbearable experience. When he obtained his prosthesis, he regained his speech and his appearance improved. Speech therapy was also of help; he felt strengthened, more independent and for a period was able to return to his life as a creative writer. The services provided by the team treating this patient—dentist, doctor, nurse, social worker, prosthodontist, speech therapist—were crucial in restoring this verbal, expressive man to a way of life so necessary to his self-esteem even for the one year which elapsed between his treatment and his death.

Patients handicapped in communication because of organic disease can be helped to maintain their socialization by encouraging them to use substitute methods—for speech, substitute body language (moving of a shoulder, tapping of the hand for signals, a nod of the head). The patient who is withdrawn because of psychological factors presents no less a challenge.

In setting a standard for oral care of the dying patient, thought should be given to the question of whether or not this standard is realistic. Where do we find these patients? They are at home, in hospitals, in nursing homes; they are ambulatory, semi-ambulatory, or bedridden. A significant proportion are not well enough to be treated in a dentist's office. Is it possible for dental mobile units to go into homes, nursing homes, terminal care facilities, even state hospitals to care for these chronically ill patients? Such a program would be costly in terms of time and personnel. Would it be prohibitive? Are adequate numbers of dentists and dental hygienists available? Are these professionals trained to work with the chronically ill? Can we find a reasonable number of personnel who have attitudes appropriate to the care of these patients? Service to terminal patients lacks some of the gratifications found in treating ambulatory, generally healthy, middle-class patients. The oral care of the patients we are talking about will often have to be closely meshed with the patients' medical and nursing care—are dentists prepared to accept these limitations?

There remains the problem of financing. What is the cost of such a program likely to be? Are third party carriers and public agencies likely to pay for this care? Will there have to be a choice between the provision of care for this patient group and more adequate dental care of our normal, healthy population? The dental profession will have to be more articulate on this subject if appropriate priorities are to be established.

In summary, oral care of the dying patient is a component part of his proper care. It is often overlooked because the treatment of the primary condition of the patient tends to take precedence over all other care. A further stumbling block is that oral care has never been acknowledged as a necessary component of general health care for all people.

Comprehensive care of the terminally ill will help to prolong the patient's productive life and help preserve his social identity. Social work is vitally concerned with the establishment of the standards of comprehensive care since it is the task of the social worker to maintain the family structure during this time of crisis and assist the patient to function as an integrated individual for as long as possible.

To provide an adequate standard of oral care for terminally ill patients there must be a marked increase of personnel and resources allocated to meet these needs. In the long run, the dental profession will play an essential role in the decision that this goal is worthwhile.

The Social Worker's Role in Care of the Dying

Constance Lamb* and Elizabeth R. Prichard**

How wisely and effectively to help the patient is a challenge to all helping professions, and of greatest significance at the time of ultimate crisis when the patient can no longer function on his own and the family unit must be helped to cope with the impending crisis. Medical personnel have concentrated their energies on the problem of maintaining life and until recently have tended to shy away from or simply deny the problems of dying and death.

In many communities and cultures where there are no organized medical and social services, it is the kindly neighbor who helps to bring a child into the world, care for the sick, tend the dying and sit with the bereaved family. Our forebears always rose to their neighbor's crisis and, to some extent, people still do act to help one another in crises. But as people have become more mobile and urbanized, families and friends are scattered, and dependence on the family or groups of neighbors has changed. Furthermore, each individual is so beset with the increased tensions of technological living that there is little left of his depleted energy to give to his neighbor. "We have witnessed more fundamental change in the way people live and in the nature of their society during this century than in all previous history!" (1)

We are a youth-oriented culture, and despite a high toll of death among the young, due primarily to accidents, the young do not envisage nor accept death. At the other end, we have an increased number of elderly persons living longer: "tens of thousands born in the 1870's and 1880's live today" (2).

---

*Supervisor of Social Work. Department of Surgery. The Presbyterian Hospital in the City of New York, Columbia-Presbyterian Medical Center, New York, New York.

** Assistant Professor, Department of Medicine (Medical Social Service), College of Physicians and Surgeons, Columbia University, New York, New York; Director of Social Service, The Presbyterian Hospital in the City of New York.

This discussion of terminal care will focus on the sociologic aspects as the social worker is confronted by them. For how social workers function in helping the dying patient is very much affected by the life styles emerging from our culture. Today, as the individual seeks to survive as an individual and not as a computerized numeral, he reaches out to be part of a group, and through the group or community re-identify himself as an individual.

The changes in society have affected the family, the relationships within the family and the emergence of certain peer groups in more influential roles within the culture. The individual's place in society traditionally has emanated from his place within the family structure. Social work has based its practical applications on the sociology, economics, anthropology, psychology and psychiatry of the cultures it is concerned with and has striven to combine its knowledge of all of these for use in a structured helping process; within the hospital setting, the effects and interactions of illness are added to these other determinants.

Because social work is problem oriented and reality focused, its concerns are the problems of daily living, of environmental pressures and the coping mechanisms of inner psychic forces. Societal changes are forcing an enlargement of our role as we are once again the "helpful neighbor" at the time of a person's greatest crisis—death. We have now the advantage of the tremendous body of knowledge which gives us new understandings of motivation, the role of the ego, breakdown of the defenses, and so on. Our concern is how to use this knowledge effectively while we help individuals in the crisis of death; but with this comes the responsibility for helping these individuals face life. One cannot help the individual face death if he has not been helped to live; both require recognition of man's material wants and inner needs. "One may also very much agree that the fear of death is in reality related to the fear of life. A person who has been able to live life with a modicum of fear and a maximum of relativity is generally able to face the fact that death may be a finite end and can be faced with dignity" (3).

Illness is a threat—a threat to one's functioning and relationships, and eventually to life itself. Thus, one starts with the problems resulting from illness. The social worker is in an advantageous position to help the patient to deal with problems which he cannot handle himself. Children must be cared for, an aged spouse looked after, income must be assured, rent must be paid. The patient who is seriously ill, yet not aware of or denying death, still has hope and this must be sustained as long as he wants it to be sustained.

The patient must be allowed to control his own affairs for as long as possible. The patient who needs assurance that someone is readying his garden for the winter is perhaps fretting because he cannot do it himself, but he is also adhering to his own yearly timetable of living. It is the patient's own timetable of life and responsibilities which should be continued as long as he is physically able and emotionally slanted. "If we can influence the family's attitude, we can serve the patient whose capacity to adapt to his illness may be inadequate. Attitudes and emotional states are contagious" (4).

Social Work Role

The primary characteristics of social work in the care of the terminal patient are: 1) it is both individual and family oriented; 2) it permits and enables continuing relationships while the patient is in the hospital, at home or in another facility; 3) its personnel have a knowledge of community resources and long-established working relationships with these resources; 4) it provides leadership in establishing these resources; 5) it has co-responsibility for continued planning of terminal care programs; 6) it is knowledgeable about and prepared to provide reality needs with sensitivity and feelings for the individual and the family, and with understanding of the psychological needs of each family member. The latter is the most constructive aspect of the social worker's role and unique to social work.

Social work is in the enviable position of having programs to offer the patient and his family which are related to urgent problems of living. The link between these problems of living and the individual's anxieties and concerns is very close, and thus, the relationship between the social worker and the patient and/or the family must be fortified by compassion and understanding.

The Patient

To help the individual, one must first understand him, what he is like as a person, his concerns for himself and his concerns for his family. What is his self-image? Does he have strong dependency needs? How has he coped with crisis in the past? Does he have meaningful spiritual values and religious ties? The patient's achievements and/or failures are often voiced at this time to the physician, nurse, clergyman, social worker; and when there is no one with whom he has a close relationship—to other patients

(5). Often, these are the clues to us that the patient realizes that this may be the end of his life. It is not infrequent for the patient to be aware, although not fully accepting, of the fact that his course will be a downhill one, and request help of the physician, nurse or social worker in making the family understand. The physician may ask for the social worker's opinion about which member of the family seems to have the strength to handle necessary responsibilities of planning for the patient.

The social worker may know a patient and his family at an early phase of an illness, months or even years before it becomes terminal. This is not uncommon in a clinic or hospital setting. Relationships are established and cemented early in the course of treatment and the patient and his family naturally turn to the social worker with social and personal concerns. The core and basis of establishing such a relationship requires full involvement and participation of all concerned, and a sharing of feelings and concerns. The troubled person needs care and understanding. Thus, when patient and family are known to the social worker for a period of time, feelings, attitudes and reactions may be foreseen, and the problems to be dealt with can more readily be determined.

In many instances after a medical diagnosis of terminal illness is confirmed, the patient and/or his family may be referred to Social Service for help. This is not an easy assignment and requires delicate handling. The social worker's own philosophy about death is of particular significance in establishing their relationship.

There are inherent difficulties in entering a case situation when a patient does not know that he is dying. The case work relationship generally is established on the basis of full participation of the patient. When the social worker enters into the situation prior to the patient's full knowledge or acceptance of the long-range goals, she may feel the burdens that such a situation imposes. The problems of everyday life must be resolved and long-range goals established without the patient being a full partner in the planning. However, this patient is assured that there is someone who will not desert him and who is involved with the things which must be done.

The Family

The initial step of the social worker is to become well acquainted with the patient and also the family members, if there are any. How the patient and family have met problems of illness previously, how stable the group is, how stable and close the parent's relationships are, what social and economic problems loom ahead, are questions which must be investigated. From experience we know that the unstable family will tend to fall apart at the first sign of a threatening illness. The stable family will rally and pull together at a time of crisis, but over a long period of time the stresses and strains can be very wearing, and sustained help from the social worker is needed. The social worker has a great deal to contribute. Medical treatment and management of the patient can be effective only if the patient is as free from personal and family conflicts as possible.

The social worker is responsible for helping to work out plans in accordance with the medical recommendations and the patient's wishes, enlisting the participation of relatives and at the same time helping the relatives experience the same sequence of reactions to the crisis as the patient (6). Sensitive awareness and full support are necessary; the social worker must be someone on whom to lean. While other hospital personnel provide this support at different stages of the illness, it is the social worker who carries this role for a more sustained and longer period. She often acts to involve the family in constructive, therapeutic behavior—maintaining the household, caring for the children, continuing the daily chores that keep a family functioning. It is a time when relationships are fully tested.

> In the case of Mrs. M., an elderly woman who had a lingering illness, the emotional dependence of her eldest daughter who was a married woman in her forties and the mother of four, presented an unusual challenge for the social worker. It was the daughter, Mrs. G., who was the closest to her mother, who visited her every day, took care of personal laundry, brought her things, and so on, and who was first told of her mother's impending terminal stage. Mrs. G. withheld this from her siblings for some time because of her own need to deny her mother's illness. She stated that she was fearful that they could not handle their feelings. With the social worker's assistance she was able to analyze her own feelings and see how they were obstacles to the care her mother needed. By accepting the reality of the situation and the social worker's support, Mrs. G. was able to mobilize her energies and to embark on a more suitable adaptive pattern in her own life. The social worker's intervention and continued support was a solace to the patient who had some awareness of her daughter's over-dependence upon her.

Many patients do not have families or close friends. Some families are so scattered that ties almost have been severed. Many of the elderly are the last remaining members of formerly large families. Some patients' families are so beset by their own problems and responsibilities that they cannot mobilize their physical and psychic energies to help. For these cases the social worker can be of great help. Much can be accomplished when assistance and support are given by someone who understands. When there is no family, the social worker must carry major responsibility for all planning.

Helping the Patient

> When Mr. B. learned that he was dying, he expressed the wish that his former wife, from whom he had been divorced many years and with whom he had had no contact since the divorce, handle his affairs. The ex-wife was happily married and living at a distance. The social worker made her first contact by letter to help Mrs. H. prepare herself and then planned to follow up by a telephone call, and so stated in the letter. Mrs. H. called back before the worker could call her to say that she would come and remain for whatever time was necessary. She came with the full knowledge and understanding of her husband. As soon as affairs were settled, the patient died—at peace. The former wife handled the matter with compassion and understanding.

Helping a patient maintain his equilibrium to whatever degree he can and communicating to him in every way possible the assurance that he will not be abandoned, are perhaps the most important aspects of helping and caring. Involved are listening to his fears, caring for his problems, respecting his individuality and providing for his needs as they arise. Recognition of the individual's inner strengths is particularly important as the following case illustrates.

> Mrs. B., a very frail, very alert 74-year-old widow with metastatic carcinoma and a grave prognosis, carefully avoided asking the doctor about either diagnosis or prognosis. She quietly declined both radiotherapy and referral to Social Service for further planning of her care. A niece who lived nearby was allowed to bring her her meals but not to seek outside help in the home.
>
> Almost two months later, Mrs. B., although all but too frail to walk unassisted, quietly came alone to Social Service. In a most dignified manner, she explained that she had not long to live and that she wanted certain information so that she could put her affairs in order. She felt the time was approaching when she should consider the specialized hospital suggested by the doctors. How would it be paid for? Would this affect her small pension? If she improved, would she be allowed to go home? If she passed away there, would her own wishes and arrangements for burial be respected? What was our honest opinion of the place she would be going to? Her main concern was that she should make this decision herself and arrange her affairs accordingly. She signed her own application to the specialized hospital and had her niece accompany her there several weeks later. She continued to lose weight but otherwise had some symptomatic relief. She then asked to be allowed to return to her apartment. Permission was given with the understanding that they would send for her if she felt the need to return. She waited until she was in extreme discomfort and then sought readmission. Shortly thereafter, she died in the terminal care hospital.

Throughout her illness, Mrs. B. quietly affirmed the acceptance of death as an inevitable part of living. The issue was not so much care in the home versus care in a hospital. The real issue for Mrs. B. was being granted the dignity inherent in making her own decisions and having them respected. Given a difficult situation, she retained her dignity by making her own determination as to the best course to follow, and when.

Meaning of Relationship

A sustained relationship and assurance that he will not be abandoned is often a "life line" for the patient. For one patient, the social worker's name and telephone number were etched in her mind when she could seemingly remember little else and it was the worker's name and number that she gave to others who sought to be of help to her.

Mrs. P., a 49-year-old former model and secretary, divorced shortly after the birth of her one child, later had been abandoned by her fiance following a radical mastectomy. When the social worker first visited her eleven months prior to her death, she had had several series of radiotherapy, had lost one eye, but had refused further palliative procedures. She was without any means of support other than periodic small loans from friends, was being evicted from a too expensive hotel apartment, did not know the whereabouts of her adolescent daughter, was eating irregularly and often postponed the filling of prescriptions urgently needed. Accustomed to a comfortable if not luxurious standard of living, she had resisted repeated efforts to refer her for public assistance and Medicaid. She was concerned about her financial situation but unable to focus on what needed to be done. Actually, she was too preoccupied emotionally to be able to move effectively on her own. She was preoccupied with the loss and rejections implicit in the abandonment by her fiance and her suppressed anger in relation to it. In addition, there was a persistent rumination on death pre-dating the malignancy and related to her mother's death from cancer of the breast when our patient was ten years of age. Psychiatric consultation had confirmed the presence of suicidal ideation but also the low probability of an actual event. She subsequently, when quite depressed, refused to accept a psychiatric admission, feeling that she "wanted to be free."

Given these circumstances, the worker's goal was to engage the patient in an effort to ameliorate her social situation without too great a threat to her ego—public assistance represented rejection and failure—and to help her make more consistent use of the medical care available to her, including the prompt filling of any prescription given her. The social worker's program of care was that of consistent availability and the gradual building up of a relationship that was both sympathetic and realistic. The worker quickly learned that Mrs. P. could not tolerate regular appointments but could tolerate a planned "haphazard" pattern. She was encouraged to pour out her grief and anger at having been abandoned. She was encouraged to talk about her fear of dying, but repetitious rumination on her mother's death over thirty years and many medical events ago was not encouraged. The resistance to the essential application for public assistance was eased when the worker accompanied the patient for the first interview. She had trouble complying with Department of

Social Service regulations— e.g., that she keep those in authority informed of her frequent changes of address, but eventually she learned to cope with their demands on her own. In specific emergencies, the worker occasionally supplied small amounts of cash but kept this to the minimum since it did not really solve the problem, tended to make Mrs. P. feel guilty and, in any event, the Department of Social Service was the basic resource, however limited it might be.

As she established a firmer relationship with the worker, the tendency to ruminate on her mother's death diminished and was converted into expressions of her embittered feelings when her father remarried. She came to the realization that some of these had been childhood fantasies, not really related to the actual people involved. She began to speak more about fearing her own death and the somewhat varying responses of the different physicians whom she had pressed for information. At one point she asked for placement information about "somewhere that people go to die," where she could work "until her time came"; she was reassured when she was told that a move of this sort would not be possible. She then began to clock off the months she had succeeded in living beyond the year's time given by one physician. She eventually found an attending physician in the clinic whom she regarded as her personal physician and from whom she derived great reassurance when he responded to her questions one time by telling her he honestly did not know the answers. She felt better, slept better and began a more purposeful search for a small apartment. She made renewed efforts to locate her daughter, who had called the social worker with the idea that they might find a place to share. They were in a hotel room together when she abruptly developed neurological symptoms that resulted in her final hospitalization.

Over the eleven month period, there were many times when neither the social worker nor the friends to whom she had given the worker's name and telephone number, knew where Mrs. P. was currently staying. She had lost most of her possessions, or pawned them, or left them at someone's apartment for safe-keeping. The only consistent feature in her wandering, often while quite depressed, was that she remembered how to reach the worker and did this in lieu of contacting her next of kin. Friends called. Passing acquaintances, hotel owners and restaurant keepers called. All were concerned and some were frightened by her appearance and what she had told them of her plight. Often they offered some small help such as a few nights' lodging.

When the social worker visited the patient in a nearby city hospital, she had a passing loss of speech but startled the floor staff with her instant recognition of her visitor. On the social worker's last visit, Mrs. P. immediately started to discuss the problems of everyday living; whether to let The New York City Department of Social Services know where she was, what to do about a pawn ticket due to expire, and how to reach her daughter. It was as though she associated the worker with the difficult task of coping with living one day at time, something she wanted to hang onto for as long as she could. To this patient whose life had been a series of rejections, another's acceptance of her as an individual had great meaning.

Sustaining life on its course of everyday living is a challenge to the patient whose condition and symptoms are constant and preoccupying reminders of illness, fear of dying and abandonment, even while he is still able to remain in the community.

Mrs. C., a 66-year-old widow living alone, was referred to Social Service for transportation to out-patient radiotherapy treatments. Her diagnosis was squamous cell epithelium of the base of the tongue. There was a brief readmission that indicated no recurrence but she continued for many months to mention how distressed she was by dryness of the mouth. Adequate food intake had been further hampered by illfitting old dentures, now scheduled for replacement in the near future. There was a history of neurological and cardiac problems but the patient's greatest concern had been the oral discomfort.

Originally, there was some thought of placing her in a nursing home but a home visit showed a good apartment in an elevator building and a telephone at the bedside. It was felt she might do better there, given some help in the home and some sustained, supportive help with the cooperation of community agencies. Her capable part-time housekeeper now breaks the isolation and takes care of the heavier household tasks and helps the patient get to her clinic appointments.

Mrs. C. attached a special significance to some delays on the new dentures, taking it to mean there was something the Dental Clinic knew and did not want to tell her, i.e., that she had a recurrence of the cancer or was expected to have one and that they therefore did not think her life expectancy warranted the expenditure of funds and effort on her behalf. Sharing these ideas with the worker was helpful up to a point but new dentures would obviously have considerable meaning for her.

The above illustrates a recurring problem. For many there is no source of funds, or the patient is hesitant to draw from limited savings. The patient even with a very small income and limited savings may be ineligible for Medicaid. Medicare does not meet the cost of dentures. Cost of dentures and prosthetic devices are high and funds from Social Service are limited. While it is recognized that proper dentition helps in maintaining the patient's nutrition and in sustaining the patient's image, there must also be recognition of the fact that for many, particularly older persons, life's satisfactions are limited and oral satisfactions are compensatory. When a prognosis is poor, the decision to use limited funds is a difficult one. The meaning to the patient, the medical recommendations and the already established commitment to a total plan of helping should be the determining factors.

Helping a patient live with cancer over a long period is a special kind of challenge. Mrs. M., a woman in her late 30s, has an unsightly disfigurement of the right side of her face as the result of surgery for a malignancy. She refused further surgery as a corrective measure because complete rehabilitation could not be assured. Radiotherapy treatments were effective in control of metatases. Her resulting depression was an added overlay on an essentially depressed personality.

The mother of two children, both in their teens. Mrs. M. had been divorced for many years. Difficulties in bringing up the children were aggravated by her appearance, and her feelings about this in turn heightened an already basic problem in personal relationships. Referred to the psychiatry department, Mrs. M. was not amenable to continuing psychiatric treatment but did accept referral to the psychiatric social worker.

Through this relationship over a period of time, she gradually was able to accept vocational training, obtain employment, and find satisfaction in her work. When a fire destroyed her belongings she was able to find satisfaction in refurnishing the apartment. She involved herself in this with great vigor. Sustained encouragement, however, was very much needed through all the steps she took in this. Furthermore, through counseling sessions the social worker was able to encourage the patient to recognize her children's needs and to strengthen her own role as mother. The children were sent to camp for a few summers with the help of Social Service funds, since both mother and children needed rest and relaxation from one another, and the opportunity to develop their separate identities.

Helping a patient to maintain his self-image requires sensitivity and readiness to respond. The patient's ability to manage disfigurement is dependent upon his own inner security and methods of coping. When patients are aware of how unsightly they appear and how troubled they are about this, they should be encouraged to explore all possible means to improve their appearance.

Mr. R., a tall, heavy-set 69-year-old truck driver with angiosarcoma of the scalp, metastatic to the lung, was referred to Social Service for help in obtaining a wig. On Social Security and pensions, he lacked the funds to purchase this for himself and was angry that Medicaid would not provide it. He was "fed up" with the ill-concealed reactions of some of his relatives to the unsightly scar tissue on his bald spot and ear. Basically a jovial, gregarious person, he now avoided family gatherings and church because he did not feel he could remove the cap he wore pulled down as far as possible.

Mr. R. bluntly told the worker he did not think she, or Medicaid, or anyone else would find him worth helping with anything that cost as much as the wig since we knew and he knew he had cancer and had only a short time to live. When he was encouraged to talk about his prognosis, he revealed that he did not think too much about it but that he felt life was a gamble anyway and he probably had more time left than his doctors and his relatives thought he did. He felt his own robustness and ability to "take it" were what had carried him through several surgical procedures and he was ready to gamble on more, if need be. His own immediate goal was to lessen his isolation.

Once the patient's own assessment of the threat posed by his illness was clear and open between patient and worker, it was not too difficult to find some release through action: shopping for the best wig and making a careful survey of resources that might be helpful to other patients;

involving his adult children by having them contribute what would have been spent on his birthday and Christmas presents, discussing with his wife what they could manage from their pension, and letting Social Service also add a relatively small gift. The result was a sense of confidence and accomplishment for the patient, a feeling that he could still take the initiative to act on certain aspects of his problem and that he did not have to resign himself passively to social isolation.

Interdisciplinary Relationship

It is imperative that the social worker be in close communication with the physician, nurse and other members of the clinical team. As anxieties mount on the part of the patient and family there is need for a well-defined team approach. While the patient is in the hospital, the social worker's responsibilities may be focused primarily on the family. If the patient is to be transferred, then the social worker should act directly to establish a relationship with the patient to help him establish independence from the hospital.

Patients and families may resist the idea of transfer from the hospital and anxiety and anger emerge when they are faced by impending loss and an apparent rejection by the hospital. These feelings can be handled by channeling them into realistic, sound plans for the benefit of the patient. It is the social worker who has the primary responsibility for carrying out transfer plans and who must provide the patient and family with continuous support. Full involvement of the physician and nurse also is necessary as preparations for separation from the hospital are finalized. Sensitivity on everyone's part is essential.

Planning for the Terminally Ill Patient

The increased emphasis on use of hospital beds for the acutely ill patient has made more visible the lack of suitable and sufficient resources for the terminally ill patient. Societal attitudes towards death, the reluctance to recognize the needs of the dying patient, and the meaning and effect of death on the family are reflected in the community by its lack of preparation in providing patient care services for the terminally ill patient and his family.

Whether the patient is to be cared for at home in a nursing home or a terminal care facility depends upon the medical recommendations and extent of care the patient needs, his family relationships, the wishes of the patient and family, and the availability of resources. A limited, all too limited, number of facilities under voluntary auspices are geared to the care of the terminally ill patient.

Care at home is valid when an important consideration is to keep patient and family together as long as possible. Nursing services and supervision of patient care by the Visiting Nurse Association, and homemaker and other services provided by Cancer Care and the American Cancer Society, have enabled many patients to remain at home. These services, developed and expanded in recent years, at first met much resistance to their contention that very sick people can be cared for at home. Some hospitals have home care programs which provide effective service. Social workers must be constantly alert to manage the effects of emotional and physical strain on the individual and family members and to give emotional support.

We know that a great need exists for more resources for the terminally ill patient, but we do not know how extensive this need is. Efforts to obtain support for a comprehensive survey have thus far been unsuccessful. With increased interest in the concept of total care, a study is now a possibility.

The extent of the need for and range of services can best be achieved by a survey of some magnitude among hospitals, physicians, visiting nurses, families, and so on. The study can have validity only if a basis of measurement can be formulated, and this requires the combined thinking of all the professional disciplines who have not only a responsibility for patient care but also a reservoir of knowledge. Although this combined knowledge has not been fully studied and documented, there is nevertheless emerging sufficient data on which to proceed, apply, and test.

It is imperative that every effort be made to increase the number of community resources, and to apply our basic knowledge. But first, the community, in its largest sense, needs help in facing the issue directly and in uncovering its fears, anxieties and guilt so that the dying patient will not be considered expendable, and bereaved and often shattered lives can be helped during the period of adjustment which follows the death of a significant family member.

The Bereavement

Continuity of the helping relationship at the time of bereavement is of particular importance and is the final step in helping the individuals or family members most affected by the death of the patient. Gradual preparation for the transfer of roles and assumption of new responsibilities, if required, will have been started earlier. The social worker is in a unique position to be the one to encourage this preparation. Understanding of the extent of the emotional investment which an individual has in his relationship to the dying person, as well as the meaning of separation, is most important. The age of the individual and his relationship to the person who has died are also determining factors in the bereaved's reaction. In some instances, the personal loss may be very great; in others, it may be a release from an unhealthy or unsatisfying relationship, or a physically and emotionally exhausting relationship. Society does not condone a frank admission of reactions other than sorrow and thus the burden can be very difficult for those who do not feel it. The need for a therapeutic relationship with someone who knows and understands is particularly necessary to lessen and, hopefully, to eliminate feelings of guilt.

Sorrow and sadness are very personal matters and each person must cope with this in his own way. The fear that one might intrude on the individual's sorrow often results in abandonment at the time when help is needed most. Simply to be available may be sufficient. But the care of children or other family members must be maintained until the bereaved again can assume responsibility. Anger may be very much in evidence and must be understood. Emotional support must be given to those who will carry increased responsibilities. It is a period of adjustment and time is needed. Practical matters must be handled and, if necessary, the social worker must help the bereaved to mobilize his energies to do this.

Knowledge and understanding of religious/spiritual and cultural values and customs and their meaning to the bereaved are vital for the social worker. Many of our old customs are being evaluated and, no doubt, new ones will take their place. Man in each culture has shown need for these and they may well be part of the "mysterious legacies which lie within us (7)." Death is inevitable and final, and it is the end of life to which we must help the bereaved address themselves. The acuteness of sorrow can pass and whatever was meaningful in the relationship can be the basis for an enriching and sustaining force in facing the challenges of everyday living.

References

1. R. Clark, *Crime in America*, New York: Simon and Schuster, 1970, p. 29.

2. *Ibid*, p. 32.

3. C. W. Wahl, In paper presented at Joint Sessions of the Medical and Psychiatric Social WorkSections at the Eighty-Sixth National Conference on Social Welfare, San Francisco, California, May, 1959. (One of three papers later published by the National Association of Social Workers, entitled, "Helping the Dying Patient and His Family," New York; 1960.)

4. P. H. Brauer, "Emotional Impact of Terminal Illness," paper presented at Symposium on a Constructive Approach to Terminal Illness, National Cancer Foundation (now Cancer Care), New York, 1958.

5. Well described in *The Cancer Ward*, A. Solzhenitsyn, New York: Dial Press, 1968.

6. E. Kubler-Ross, *On Death and Dying*, New York: Macmillan Co., 1969.

7. R. Ardrey, *The Social Contract*, Toronto: McClelland and Stewart, Ltd., 1970, p. 30. (Published also by Atheneneum Publishers, New York, 1970.) See also pp. 27-30, "Elephant Story."

Pastoral Care of Patients with Oral Cancer

*Rev. Robert B. Reeves, Jr.**

Clergymen are not likely to see many patients with cancer in the oral cavity for several reasons. First, relative to the total number of a clergyman's parishioners, such patients are usually few and far between. Second, few patients with oral disease are inclined to think of their illness in terms of need for pastoral attention. Third, pastoral work with such patients is usually so awkward as to lead both clergyman and parishioner to avoid each other.

The patient's disinclination or reluctance to seek pastoral care has many causes, depending on the nature and severity of the disease condition.

In cases where relatively simple surgery is required, as in extraction of teeth or excision of small tumors, the threat to life or to the integrity of body-image is not extensive or vivid enough for the patient to feel in mortal danger. He is temporarily inconvenienced and suffers a limited amount of pain, but normal healing and dentures rather quickly restore him to a sense of well-being. What conscious feelings he has about malignant disease are usually expressed as embarrassed annoyance at the inconvenience. This is especially true when he loses his teeth. Underneath, however, he may be very much afraid. But the fear, as fear, is inaccessible at this level of affliction. To call for the pastor, when the trouble is only a matter of annoyance or embarrassment, would seem silly.

The pastor, too, would probably feel similarly. He might show some degree of sympathy, especially if he himself had had a similar experience, and be quite understanding of the patient's tendency to avoid contact with other people during the period of his oral inconvenience. But it would hardly occur to him to make of this an occasion for counseling or prayer. Much more likely, he would look for an opportunity to josh the patient about his "choppers" or his inability to talk for a day or two.

Nevertheless, a situation such as this does present a need for pastoral care. In the voluntary association of any religious group, the way a person

---

* Chaplain, The Presbyterian Hospital in the City of New York, Columbia—Presbyterian Medical Center, New York, New York.

presents himself is a matter sometimes of preoccupying concern. The kind and degree of participation in the activities of the group depend in large part on the image a person feels he is projecting. Very few people, for example, will attend church during the period between loss of teeth and the fitting of dentures; or while they may slip in and out of worship service unobtrusively, they will shun church suppers or other social occasions. If the pastor calls on them in home or hospital during such a period, he is likely to hear embarrassingly profuse apology for their appearance or indistinct speech. They convey a sense of damage to self-image, and it seems to make them want to hide.

So, while neither the patient nor the pastor may think it is very important, pastoral attention at such a time can be very meaningful. The pastor's acceptance of the patient, just as he is, minus teeth and with garbled speech, goes a long way to dispel the patient's feeling of isolation. While neither counseling nor prayer may be indicated, fellow-feeling is greatly needed. A pastor who takes the time to "be with" such patients may find their gratitude out of all proportion to the actual time involved, and their readiness for pastoral care much deepened when the disease becomes worse.

When the disease requires more severe surgery or radiotherapy, or when a tracheotomy becomes necessary to maintain an airway, the patient is much more likely to feel in danger. While permanent disfigurement may not as yet be in the picture, the surgeon knows that it may eventually become necessary, and the patient consciously begins to fear it. He usually has, however, so much immediate discomfort and mechanical difficulty that his attention is pretty well taken up, and the fear of disfigurement is crowded to the background.

The immediate trouble is bad enough, especially when mucous must be suctioned from the trachea. The sensation is unlike anything the patient has ever felt before, and accompanying sounds at first are terrifying. I have found very few patients who were prepared for the experience, and many who panicked when mucous suction first had to be applied. When the suction tube is inserted through the mouth, gagging usually results. The skill and alertness of nurses vary greatly; an awkward or too-vigorous application of the tube can give the patient a dreadful fright; delay in its application, when mucous impedes breathing, can quickly bring on panic. The cavalier attitude often displayed by staff is no great help at such a time. The patient may feel he is within an inch of suffocating, his life depends on their alertness and skill, and he wants the staff to take his danger seriously.

Later on, when he is a little more used to the sensation and the sound, he may get over some of his fright. The most reassuring thing is for him to learn to suction himself, so that he is not dependent on others, and can himself control the thrust of the tube. Once he knows that he himself can take adequate care of his trachea, he settles down to it as if he had been doing it all his life, and thinks nothing of using a tube in the course of visits from family, friends and clergy.(If anything, he tends to make it sound a little worse, just for their benefit!)

Communication, of course, is a great problem. Until he has healed enough to permit a plug in the tracheal opening, or a finger over it, the patient cannot talk. He may at first try sign language with his hands, but finds people so stupid at interpreting what he wants, that he quickly turns to writing his messages. This is very limiting, because of the time and quantities of paper that it requires, and his own ineptness at expressing himself in writing. So the messages tend to be minimal and concerned chiefly with his basic physical needs and the mechanics of his care. People who ask him questions that cannot be answered with a hand sign, a shake of the head, or a brief written word become annoying to him. At the very time when his dependent condition makes personal support a necessity, his inability to communicate tends to shut him off in isolation. He wants to say so much more than he can comfortably write that he becomes frustrated, sometimes furious, and often then depressed. Visitors are usually a trial. Fellow-patients in the same four- or five-bed room hardly ever communicate with one another.

Such a patient seldom calls for clergy in the immediate postoperative period because he is so preoccupied with the mechanics of survival, and later, because communication is so difficult. If pastoral attention is requested, it is probably by the family, who are usually scared out of their wits by the first sounds of suctioning they hear; or if they call for a pastor before surgery, it is because they are so much more aware than the patient permits himself to be, of the possibility of disfigurement.

The essential thing in a pastor's attention to such a patient is that it be undemanding. This does not mean that a pastoral monologue should be delivered. It means, rather, that a pastor be comfortable with silence, content in few words to express his concern and support, make simple inquiries that can be answered with a nod or gesture, sit for a few minutes, and leave—but come back often. Prayer may or may not be indicated. But a word that the pastor will remember the patient in prayer is never amiss. The patient will show when he is ready for more extended "conversation" by reaching for his writing pad and volunteering information. Much of such "talk," I find, is matter-of-fact, with little disclosure of inner feeling; almost always hopeful, with great pleasure shown in small gains; and with rarely a reference to the possibility of eventual disfigurement. Complaints, if expressed at all, seem to center on the nuisance of tube feeding, if that is necessary, or on the limitation to activity imposed by dependence on the suction hose.

When radical, disfiguring surgery is performed, and the voice box or part of the jaw or a cheekbone must be cut away, both patient and pastor find the going very rough. Sometimes doctors cannot tell the patient fully what they are going to do, because they themselves do not know before surgery is under way; or they tell him in words he does not fully understand; or they tell him clearly but he blocks it out of his awareness: it is too awful to think about, and denial comes to the rescue. In any case, the patient rarely has a clear idea of the extent of the damage that is going to be done to him. Before such surgery, few patients ask for a pastor; and if the pastor goes to them, he is likely to think them stoical or numb, denial working overtime to blot out what would otherwise be grievous beyond bearing.

The state that such a patient may be in following surgery can sometimes fill even the most experienced hospital chaplain with dismay. Part of the patient's face may be gone. Bandages and dressings may be soaked with blood and mucous. The patient appears enmeshed in tubes, drains, catheters, bottles, pumps and other equipment. Rattling gurgles issue from his windpipe. His doctors see him as little as they can and still keep track. The nurses are brisk, efficient, and very busy. His family are aghast and try not to show it—very unconvincingly. Long before the patient gets his courage up to take a sneak look at himself in a mirror, he reads the signals of the people around him, that he is horrible. Maybe an aide or orderly puts a hand on his shoulder in passing, but all in all, it is a terrible and lonely experience.

To all the other nightmare aspects of such mutilating surgery may be added odor, the distinctive and nauseating odor of cancer. Patients seem always to be aware of it, if not through their own olefactory sense, then through the involuntary hints of repugnance they see in those who attend them. To the patient's feeling of isolation, caused by his inability to talk and the tendency of staff to avoid or treat him impersonally, is added the feeling of being so offensive to others as to be beyond acceptance. He feels shunned, abandoned, walled off in a pit of stinking misery. Depression is the inevitable result.

Here, probably more than in any other condition of disease, the patient needs someone to reach through the misery to reclaim him as a human being. Sometimes, but rather rarely, a physician, nurse, or family member may be able to do it. Somehow, a pastor must. I confess, however, that this is the most difficult kind of experience I have to face in my duties as a chaplain. I dread seeing such patients. But I go. I go and I sit with them for a little while. And I put my hand on them, and say very little. But I go often, and keep alert for signs that the depression may be lifting. For the depression does lift, the will-to-live revives, the mechanics of survival require the patient's attention, and there comes a day— not more than several days after surgery usually—when, as I approach, he lifts his head or hand in greeting. Then, I can begin to talk with him, and he can nod or gesture or write in answer. The amazing thing is how often, in answer to "How are things going?" I get the response, "I can't complain." It is two-edged, I know: "It wouldn't do any good to complain," is one part of the message; but the other is there too—"I'm OK."

What it is, I have never been able to be sure. Denial, of course, is working. But just plain raw courage is in it, too—guts. More often than not, a kind of stoic acceptance sets in, rarely cheerful, rarely glum. The patient quietly busies himself in the tasks of self-care, takes refuge within the boundaries set by his condition, seems not to fret, talks very little about the future, often giving the impression he is waiting.

I have never had a patient in this terminal period of oral cancer ask me to pray, and the times I have offered to do so, the response has usually been a noncommittal lift-of-hand or tilt-of-head, as if to say, "If it would please you, go ahead." I suspect that the damage to selfhood is so severe as to blot out any thought of a good God, and the thought of a monstrous God is so painful that it, too, is repressed. Religion, as we normally think of it, just does not figure. The issues of life and death are reduced to simple dignity and courage. It is the archaic Greek thing—holding on to what it is to be a man, under fated doom. If one can honor that and stay with him, such a patient will get the message that God does not desert him, either. That is enough. The patient need not say it, nor need anyone else.

APPENDIX

Surgical Notes:
Case of Sigmund Freud, M.D.*

In the sixteen years during which Professor Pichler attended Freud he kept regular notes of the case, every visit being recorded and the details entered with an admirable exactitude. For months at a time there would be daily interviews, so hard was it to relieve the discomfort in the wound. The notes were made in a variation of the Gabelsberger system of stenography invented by Pichler's father and so were unintelligible to other people. After his death there was only one person who could decipher them, his old secretary. The indefatigable Max Schur, to whom Pichler had left his notes on his death, sought her out and persuaded her to undertake the laborious task of transcribing them: this in spite of the difficulty that all the medical expressions were indicated only by abbreviations. Even so the notes occupy fifty-three foolscap sheets of close type. They give an unforgettable picture of the long drawn out distress, or even agony, through which Freud passed in those years.

Dr. Lajos Levy has been good enough to translate these notes into English, and Dr. Schur has checked the translation from his personal knowledge of the details. I have made a small selection of them, mainly for their medical interest, and append them here. But they can give little idea of the day-to-day struggle, by the countless manipulations and applications, to procure some relief for the continual discomfort and pain.

Extract of Case History[a]

9/26/23   Consultation with laryngologist Hajek who operated on a papillary prolifering leukoplakia at right anterior palatinal arch last spring, excision far into healthy tissue. (Histolog. carcinoma.) Now recurrence at anterior edge of operation-site, at posterior end of superior processûs alveolaris, in form of crateriförm ulcer extending over large part of buccal mucous membrane and small part of tongue and mandible. I constructed prosthesis, then undertook on special request clearance of submandibular and cervical glands and ligature of carotis externa and, shortly afterward, resection of maxilla including anterior part of ramus ascendens mandibulae. Soft palate preserved, with posterior edge within area of scar in palatinal arch. Wound in soft tissue covered with Thiersch-graft.

11/12/23   Operation of recurrence at posterior border with removal of most of right soft palate and of processus pterygoideus. Thiersch-graft. End of Dec., 1923 Prosthesis finished. X-ray irradiations during 1923 and 1924. Since then repeated alteration of prosthesis, finally provided with springs.

11/19/25   Operation of impacted Lower Left 5 with small cyst.

1929   Patient had new prosthesis constructed by Professor Schroeder in Berlin, with drift for upper teeth, still in use now.

10/10/30   Excision of small papillary leukoplakia in operation area, Thiersch-graft.

2/7/31   Removal of new warty papilloma by diathermy.

*Appendix B. Surgical Notes, from Volume 3 of *The Life and Work of Sigmund Freud* by Ernest Jones, M.D., c 1957 by Ernest Jones, Basic Books, Inc., Publisher, New York. Permission for the inclusion of this chapter granted by Basic Books, Inc.

aSummary report sent to Exner by Pichler on Freud's departure for London.

4/23/31   Another excision and Thiersch-graft.

Sept., 1931 New attempt to have prosthesis constructed by Dr. Kazanijan from Boston. Subsequently several more prostheses.

3/7/32   Other small operations of the same kind: 7/29, 8/16, 10/6, 12/8/32, 5/16 and 9/5/33 excisions and coagulations of small papilloma. (Histolog. negative.)

1/12/34   Cauterization with caustic potash.

3/23-7/11/34 165 radium mgh. Contact-irradiations at distance of ca. 4-8 mm and 1 mm, brass filter. Has to be abandoned since patient felt that irradiations caused migraine and severe disturbances of general condition.

9/24-12/6/34 125 mgh. radium. Had to be abandoned again.

3/23/35   Destruction of small papillomata by diathermy.

4/30/35   Destruction of small papillomata by diathermy.

8/19 and 10/11/35 Destruction of brown dry keratosis by diathermy.

3/10/36   Destruction of papilloma by diathermy.

7/14/36   Excision of more elevated nodule by diathermy (histolog. findings cancer) therefore

7/18/36   deepening of wound, resection of some bone substance and thorough coagulation.

12/12/36   Coagulation of very suspect ulcer.

4/22/37   Biopsy excision of warty proliferation at site of former operation at inner wall of ramus ascendens mandibulae; evipan narcosis. (Histolog. negative.)

1/22/38   Excision of ulcerous and simultaneously raised place and thorough coagulation of focus. (Histolog. findings positive.)

2/19/38   Excision of suspect wart at site of last operation. (Histolog. negative.)

6/2/38   Last examination. In one place keratosis in form of recurrent brown crust. In several places slight papillary formations, non-suspicious according to previous experience.

Pichler Notes

1923/9/26 Consultation with Dr. Hajek. In spring he performed an excision at the right anterior arch of the palate because of a proliferative papillary leukoplakia. It had been planned as an explorative measure, but was extended far beyond the diseased parts. The histological findings were positive. After the operation no complaints. Now, in the last weeks, pains and progressive lockjaw. There is a crater-shaped typical ulcer at the posterior part of the Tub. maxillaris with slight infiltration into the palato-glossal fold continuing into the buccal mucous membrane and over the margin of the mandible. The palate itself is reduced in size by the previous operation and scarred. The surface of the hard palate at its posterior part has some protrusions. Only one submaxillary lymphatic gland is palpable, immediately behind the exterior maxillary artery. Patient makes the condition that he should not be attended as a colleague, but pay a fee.

Project: partial resection of the maxilla with block-anaesthesia and removal of a splinter of the mandible (Resectio anguli interni). Experiment on corpse demonstrates that it is possible to weaken the mandible from the buccal side by multiple piercings and by cutting with fissure-burrs until a splinter together with the coronary process up to the Incisura can be split off and the whole piece including the upper jaw bone be removed.

9/27 Cleaning of teeth. Exploration of teeth.

10/4 Operation at the Sanatorium Auersperg. Assistant: Dr. Bleichsteiner. Pantopon 0,03, Scop. 0,003, Di. 0,02, 2/3 cc. of this solution to start and 1½ cc. later; block-anaesthesia with ½% novocain into Cerv. and Lingu. nerves, angular incision. Typical clearance of the submaxillary glands and ligature of the art. carotis ext. peripherally to the artery thyreoidea sup. Two jugular and some submaxillary glands are enlarged and at cross section a little suspicious (no malignant cells on histological examination).

10/11 Operation at the Sanatorium Auersperg. Assistants: Dr. Hofer and Dr. Bleichsteiner. 1½ cc. of above mentioned solution; excellent success of block-anaesthesia: 3rd branch by oblique path, 2nd branch by Payr's method, local anesthesis of palate and lip faultless. Cut through the middle of the upper lip, then around the nose till half height. After that, broad cut around the buccal mucous membrane till Upper Right 7, exposing the Fossa canina by raspatory and separating the mucous membrane and the buccal gum at Upper Right 7-3. Then division of the masseter muscle above at the os zygomaticum, to enable it to be turned down later, to cover with it the gap at the mandible and to stitch it up to the margin of the cut palate. Then opened the jaws by Heister, detaching the sinew of the m. temporalis from the Proc. coron., extraction of Upper Right 7 and from the alveola of Lower Left 7 to the Incis. setting some boreholes obliquely from upper outside to lower inside at the mandible, linking them partly by sawing with Sudeck fraise and partly chiseled through. Then chiseled off the crista zygomatica high above, cutting around tumor from Upper Right 3 which has been extracted too, through the soft palate, the superior parts of the tonsils and the lingual mucous membrane of the mandible, chiseling through the fossa canina, the proc. pter. at its root and at the hard palate, and finally pulling forward the tumor and severing the nervus pterygoideus internus. At this point the whole piece broke up into 3 fragments: Proc. Cor., upper jaw and the tumor. At the wound side of the latter no macroscopically observable diseased tissue. No strong bleeding. Suturing the mucous membrane of the palate below to the Masseter muscle, further below to a 2 cm. broad flap which has been isolated from the buccal membrane (below up to the gum), disregarding the papilla Stenoni to create at least one unstrained bridge of mucous membrane from the palate arch over to the angulus int. Insertion of the prosthesis; the wound margin of the soft palate being drawn sidewise with two sutures below the prosthesis. Maxillary sinuses polypous but otherwise normal, mucous membrane only partly removed. Tamponed (Packed), above the tampon the deep gap between the upper and lower jaw, which partly goes into the soft palate below the mucous membrane, filled up by a Stentsclod of which anterior margin lies under the wound-surface of the cheek-flat. Thierschgraft of this Stents-clod from the left upper arm. Skin suture. The prosthesis in addition to the claps fastened also to Upper Left 1-4. Patient sleeps during the greater part of the operation. Nervus alv. inf. and lingualis may not have been injured. Perhaps the only mistake not to have removed more of the M. pter. int. Afterward pulse good, 64. Caffeine, calcium, digitalis-injection. Drip-enema.

10/12   Very slight reaction. Condition good, slept well. Pat. cannot speak. Thirst. Drip-enema.

10/13   After feeding by nasal tube, patient, who felt very weak, improved very much. Evening sudden rise of temperature to 39 (102.2) with sensation of weakness. Camphora, Digitalis, After 2 or 3 hours decrease of temperature to normal. Objectively everything all right.

11/7   Since day before yesterday increasing pain. Seems to originate from region of Proc. pt. where small irregular ulcer is visible after sloughing off necrotic tissue. Some ex-cochleation at this point. Some pus oozing from one spot. No sequestrum to be seen. Upper clod tested and prosthesis taken for vulcanisation.

11/9   UL 4 bites heavily on Proc. alv. Chiseling improves entry and removal of prosthesis. Bite satisfactory on the right but pushes upper prosthesis backward and spoils contact with neck of teeth. If tied on above, bite too high. Therefore polishing of both 3 right side and removal of UR 5-4 from prosthesis.

11/10   Again increased pain. Decreasing size of prosthesis at the point of the suspicious lesion; improvement. Stents-cast with upper prosthesis to supply it with teeth.

11/12   Received Stoerck's pathological report, visited patient, informed him, induced him to decide to be operated on the same day.

P.M.   Operation in Sanatorium Auersperg. Assistants: Dr. Hofer and Dr. Hertzka. After pantopon scopolamine,block-anaesthesia: Payr and 3rd branch into Foramen ovale. Incision at cheek-scar toward fissura oris and speculum suffices for access. Cut through soft palate ca 1½ cm from free margin, from here around tumor up to palate bone and proc. pter. Chiseling off and extracting the latter by severing the soft tissue-connections. Probably transection of nervus and arteria alv. inf. Heavy bleeding but not from major blood-vessel. After inspection of specimen, margins of which appear healthy, removal of additional piece at inferior and lingual border; kept for biopsy. Following this, insertion of a Stents-clod with Thiersch-graft, covered by prosthesis. Both sheets of soft palate sutured to each other, one of sutures joined to prosthesis. Finally, suturing of rhombic defect in the buccal mucous membrane along opposite diagonal.

11/14   Suture between soft palate and prosthesis came off, Stents-clod slipped into mouth causing great trouble. Clod shredded and removed with probable damage to Thiersch-graft.

11/19   Calls on patient on 15th, 16th, 17th. On 19th violent pain, no fever. On 17th patient underwent a Steinach-operation[b] for "rejuvenation," hoping for possible effect on cancer-predisposition. Investigation of specimens by Sternberg show only granulation tissue on two particles of the specimen, carcinoma on one side of third particle.

11/27   Lower prosthesis adjusted with black guttapercha on lower left. No pain; bite still somewhat high. Cannot understand why bite too high after having taken impressions twice. Anyway, clasp LL 4 not far enough lingually.

11/28   Bite still somewhat high but not troublesome, can remain. Lower prosthesis with clasp-supplement taken for vulcanization. Cast of upper clod with wax-extension, should be vulcanized and simultaneously extended upward and to posterior pharyngeal wall. More guttapercha added to top of upper plate and inserted with packing for enlargement of antrum.

12/10   Since prosthesis tied now only to UL 1 with some support from clasp UR 2, these teeth sensitive through overstrain. UL 1 shows movement toward lingual side since prosthesis tends to drop in this direction. Have to counteract this by occlusion on lower right; if necessary all front teeth will have to be connected by wire-gallery and used for support. Some additional guttapercha added to top of clod to provide extension into the antrum. All teeth tied, last molar extracted to lower bite. Otherwise all right. Swallowing and speech very good.

12/20   Prosthesis fits now almost perfectly, no sagging backward. Prosthesis treatment can be considered completed. Patient manages to-day to remove and re-insert all parts of prosthesis. Decision for prophylactic x-ray therapy. Consultation with Holzknecht who comes to my consulting room to examine the patient. Decides for irradiation partly with, partly without prosthesis and begins with first session immediately to-day.

1924/2/7   New prosthesis with gallery-clasp for front teeth and hook-closure, otherwise as before. Fits tighter than prosthesis No. 1, weighs less. Speech better right away. Removal and insertion easier than with No. 1.

2/11   Insertion of prosthesis 2 with closure of hinge-clasp repaired and closing-hooklet removed backward. Patient feels pressure on left upper part. speech worse.

bLigation of the spermatic duct.

2/12   Everything all right on left upper part. Speech much worse, perhaps hinge-clasp too loose. Tightened, some polishing on lower left.

2/26   Altered prosthesis fits rather well, but speech is very bad. Considerable improvement after further addition of guttapercha to back of clod.

2/28   This time clod fitted badly on lower part, not having clicked into groove on back. Has to be remoulded completely and palate-plate pressed upward and backward during insertion. Fits well after insertion but speech quite nasal.

3/6   Pain left on upper and lower part. Correction of pressure points. Otherwise, pain seems to originate chiefly from soft palate which is jammed at its cut edge ca. 2 mm in front of the uvula between posterior sharp margin of palate plate and the quasi obturating back part of the left half palate extending to guttapercha clod. Soreness caused by jamming. Rounding off posterior margin of plate, correction of pressure point. Guttapercha-supplement and clod which became separated, united again. General swelling of mucous membrane, caused possibly by "flu."

3/12   All kinds of unpleasant sensations; speech worse. Cannot find the reason. Have given more play to soft palate, especially on nasal side.

3/14   Consultation with Docent Stern[c] who finds hardly any sign of rhinolaly. Gutzmann's test a-j shows almost no difference whether nose occluded or open. Substantial subjective improvement, speech relieved since last chiseling. Some more chiseling. Now rather difficult to insert prosthesis so that it clicks into channel. Patient will have to exercize it by biting on piece of wood with upper and lower right molars.

4/10   Prosthesis taken for mending of countersunk holes. Prosthesis 1 is very poor substitute by now, has to be tied on as best possible. Repaired prosthesis 2 reinserted.

5/27   Speech worse, obviously nasal, all the more so since last modification. Supply of guttapercha at the point of uvula-channel seems to improve it. Lockjaw much improved. Also swallowing of fluids, which has been much more troublesome, seems improved.

7/1   Closure when drinking cold water worse again, therefore attempt to supply more guttapercha. Closure improved. But greatest discomfort from pressure and strain on right side for which cause cannot be found. Perhaps due to sinus trouble which is treated by Neumann. Advice to remove prosthesis more frequently to improve condition if possible.

9/30   New prosthesis 2 excellent for three days. Since then worse, coinciding with heavy cold, possibly some general swelling, no other findings. Inside prosthesis no fluids, hardly any uncleanness.

cA speech specialist.

10/6   Tension entirely gone but the disagreeable fact remains that prosthesis drops on both sides, on the left some more than on the right, creating discomfort. Only remedy would be springs which I should like to avoid as long as possible. Instead attempt to correct hold of hinge-split by supplying Kerr at front.

12/23   Pain improved but mastication and drinking worse, fluids regurgitating through nose since plate fits more loosely again. Fastening of screw by 1½ turns seems insufficient. Unless patient gets used to it, only remedy to increase supply of guttapercha on top of plate again so as to produce better adhesion. May try to fit some sort of padded bands or riders to prevent slipping of hinge-clasp toward necks of teeth. Treatment with silver nitrate of upper and lower necks of teeth repeated.

1925/2/10   Coryza improved. Some discomfort due to wobbling of prosthesis. Since tightening of screws helps only temporarily and hinge-clasp continues to mount toward neck of teeth, plan to fit knobs. First a platinum band is affixed to UR 2 with small platinum-pin, a screwed gold peg to UL 4, with corresponding holes drilled into hinge-clasp. If necessary, perhaps teeth UR 3-1/UL 1-3 to be altered similarly. Prosthesis 2 to receive the same new hinge-clasp.

3/10   UL 2-3 pulps extracted and roots filled.

3/12   UL 3 screw cemented in. Fits very well now but speech completely nasal. Therefore prosthesis inserted with guttapercha. UR 1 and perhaps UL 2 to be devitalized and then prosthesis finally adjusted to palate.

4/24   Prosthesis 3 very good for one day, then very bad again due to "hanging down of teeth right above." Seems to have come about through twisting of the knob at closure and might be remedied by tightening of screw. Screw fixed in this position with cement. Prosthesis 2 with new gold-gallery fits into place after some difficulties, but interferes with bite now considerably, has to be adjusted further.

7/5   Several good days, then very bad again. What is worst is the depressing hopelessness about the inability to do anything. Has slept eleven hours. No objective evidence except slight gingivitis, especially at lingual side of UR 2 and at papilla between UR 2-1, where gum is extraordinarily hyper-sensitive. Evidently the matter is mainly "nervous." Ablation of papilla and part of free gingiva margin by electrocautery. Orthoform and later massage.

9/9   At the incision-margin of the hard palate, toward the center of the hole leading to the nose, a circular, flat, ragged protuberance has appeared, with the mucous membrane in the vicinity perhaps more papillary than before. Area appears somewhat suspect, might mean recurrence. Worst of all is catarrh of nasal mucous membrane. Even before his operation patient suffered once or twice yearly from purulent discharges from sphenoidal and ethmoidal sinuses; was not much disturbed by these otherwise.

11/19   For five days now some sensitiveness left below; since last night swelling and pain, no sleep during night. On 17th attempt to arrest inflammation by irradiation. But Holzknecht considers operation unavoidable.
Operation in my consulting room. O. 7 Modiscop and three times 2 cc. 4% novocain mandibular and buccal. Opening of gum distally at LL 3 where it adheres strongly to bone affected by inflammatory process. Moderate quantity of pus evacuated. Curetting of granuloma of moderate size with exposure of crown of LL 5 incrusted by tartar. Further exposure of this through chiseling away of bone, finally easy extraction with elevator since tooth fairly loose. Root found to be short, enormously thickened by cement-deposits. Cyst-sac and granuloma extirpated fully. Packing.

1926/11/10 Fitting of new prosthesis 4. Impossible to insert as a whole. Fits quite well when inserted but speech gets indistinct. Bite in oral cavity rather difficult. Discussed trouble caused by unending tiresome sinus catarrhs with secretion which Laufer used to treat successfully by irrigation.

1927/6/9 Since last time patient saw Dr. Wolf twice because of paradental abscess of UL 4. Great improvement after curettage. Since apex can be reached with scaler, and since patient is on point of leaving Vienna, tooth is extracted with fingers, white guttapercha substituted for it on duplicate prosthesis. Right above further reduction of pressure-point, removal of old guttapercha.

6/27   Bad state after two days' relief with use of prosthesis 3. Again, one excellent day. Upper part a bit loose. Guttapercha bolster renewed. At point outside, where lacuna of mucous membrane was situated, blunt excision of piece (preserved); mucous membrane here at least 5 mm thick, covered toward lumen with resistant thin skin (perhaps epithelium extending over from Thiersch-graft).

7/4   Exactly the same as before; only one tolerable day after using old prosthesis for 1-2 days with manifold discomfort. Patient suggests removal of extension which protrudes into antrum. After casting for eventual restoration of status quo extension removed.

10/4   Prosthesis 4 supplied with guttapercha and vulcanized, fitted with steel-spring holders with ricochet-channel above and below.

10/18   After several alterations of springs in interval, to-day severe pain, general discomfort, pressure as if springs were too strong. Objectively noticeable that springs fail now to keep posterior part right above in place, being either too weak altogether or having working point too far frontal.

11/4   Springs of prosthesis 4 lengthened again and soldered at one point. Gold clasp of prosthesis 3 corrected further; should be tried for a longer period, may adjust itself through shrinkage of bed. New lower prosthesis is made from cast of old one. Fits well. Prosthesis 4 continues to produce "swellings" and disturbs hearing. Perhaps owing to obturation of tube.

1928/3/6   Right spring much better but not altogether comfortable. Prosthesis 5 with casted clod cannot be inserted fully and elevates bite. Stents-clod to be reduced all over by ½ cm and piece provided with vertical springs running in tubes.

3/8   Prosthesis 5 tried with vertical spring tucked into two telescope-tubes. Impossible to insert owing to lockjaw. Has to be shifted more lingually.

4/2   Tubed spring removed from prosthesis 5, on right side teeth partly removed, partly shifted more lingually, former type of spring resorted to again but further lingually. New guttapercha supplied with resultant great improvement of speech. To be used for several hours.

4/16   Everything bad. Pain at back, where swelling, sensitiveness and redness is found at posterior pharyngeal wall. Removal of guttapercha backward on upper part, some supply further below; right spring exchanged for heavy gold spring.

4/24   Prosthesis 5 cannot be used, too thick and large. Part of clod removed and replaced by shellac. Still too large. Pressure point on prosthesis 4 reduced.

5/7   Prosthesis 4 now caused pressure right below and spring interfered badly with tongue. Pressure points corrected and spring bent more outward. Prosthesis 5 handed over. It is vulcanized in one piece, hollow and closed with stopper, weighs 75 grams without springs.

1929/11/23   Patient arrives with Dr. Weinmann who attends him now, cleans prosthesis, etc., and with prosthesis made by Schroeder in Berlin. Upper teeth are joined to form compact bridge; soldered distally to this are oblique slanting slides of wide range on to which prosthesis is slipped. Prosthesis leaves left posterior half of palate uncovered, closes merely as sort of obturator. Actual clod of prosthesis seems of smaller dimensions. At present functions rather well, was still better in beginning; now variable. Only objection is risk that all pillars of upper bridge may loosen simultaneously some time and then the catastrophe would be great. Patient calls since Weinmann, and apparently also Schroeder, regard one spot as suspicious. This is an area which was marked down for some reason several years ago where mucous membrane of nose encroaches downward on palate. Nothing pathological. Perhaps swelling due to present bad coryza.

1930/10/3 Small leukoplakia behind prosthesis at palate and one place at Thiersch-graft near arch of palate where decubitus occurred; here a papillary change of surface in area of ca. 1 cm. which is suspect of precancerous proliferation of epithelium. Advice: excision and Thiersch on prosthesis. Since prosthesis not fully adjacent here, preliminary supplement of Kerr or guttapercha. One week's observation in case of spontaneous receding.

10/14 Operation: application of cedenta on prosthesis corresponding to changed area. Excision. Subjacent tissue soft and perfectly normal. Surpisingly little scar tissue. After excision more cedenta applied to fill hole completely and prosthesis pasted with several Thiersch-flaps. Diathermy-destruction of leukoplakia at edge of soft and hard palate left, near middle end of small wart-like nodule closely behind posterior margin of prosthesis left above in area of foramen palatinum. (Assistant Berg[d] and Weinmann.)

10/17 Yesterday patient had severe pain and bad night, took two veramon and pantopon, stomach upset, vomited, looks badly. Better to-day. Have resisted his wish to remove prosthesis till now but wants it so much that I decided in favor of it. Thiersch-flaps come out together with prosthesis. Hope that wound inoculated with epithelium by now. Cedenta-mass reduced and prosthesis reinserted.

[d] Pichler's private assistant.

10/18 Histological findings: small tissue piece covered over histologically with epithelium, slightly cornified in places which is prolifering to a certain depth in area described. Papillae of epithelium very deep and coarse, demarcated sharply everywhere from the substratum. This consists on the surface of rather loose connective tissue, in certain parts with chronic inflammatory infiltration; the deeper layers consist of tauter connective tissue undergoing hyaline degeneration, here without inflammatory infiltrations. No sign of malignancy. Excrescence in area of former transplantation may be due to big and coarse papillae of epithelium. Also hyaline degeneration of submucosa may have been subsidiary cause. (Report sent to Dr. Schur.)

10/18 Patient has had small broncho-pneumonia. One day fever but weakened by it and complains of pain when opening mouth which improved to-day. Supply on prosthesis removed. Wound looks all right. No obvious epithelium visible. Only orthoform prescribed.

1931/2/3 Dr. Weinmann gone abroad for one week. In the meantime patient wants to know from me: 1) why prosthesis functions so badly (rough, difficult speech, hard to understand) and 2) what wart-like protuberance at operation-site signifies. Supply of guttapercha improves condition for the moment. Protuberance is doubtless a papilloma, to be removed by electro-coagulation. Some doubts whether operation by knife would not be preferable since a suture from anterior to posterior might be established. Papilloma seems accreted with masseter or proc. pterygoideus. Lifts when contracted.

2/7   Operation: Assistant Dr. Bleichsteiner, Dr. Schur and Dr. Weinmann present. Cutting around with diathermy-knife at low current-intensity, then extirpation and coagulation of base consisting of entirely hard, infringed, tough connecting tissue; after that again thorough excochleation and again coagulation of margins. Spraying with orthoform and insertion of prosthesis.

2/13 Pain with prosthesis inserted was intolerable. Have to urge patient to tolerate prosthesis nevertheless since removal would increase later troubles. Agrees finally.

4/14 Area of diathermy epithelized for some time. But new appearance of a tumor further frontally corresponding to the scar fold protruding into mouth. Tumor is soft, irregular, partly dark colored, no longer wholly villous or velvety, has wrinkles and folds and can be shifted on underlying base. Supposedly grown fast and much. Considerable lockjaw, ca. 15 mm. Since aftereffects of diathermy operation are reported to have lasted throughout these two months, advise excision and Thiersch-graft. Guttapercha supplied to prosthesis. Patient to celebrate his seventy-fifth birthday soon, has bad coryza. Would like postponement. I advise against such long postponement. I believe soft tumor still precancerous but am against waiting (in view growth, which I have not pointed out to patient). Asked whether tumor could be left alone and malignancy risked, I advised against it. Asked whether radium or x-ray could be tried, I advise consultation with Holzknecht. The latter in sanatorium at present after operation on hand. Discussion with Dr. Schur over the telephone.

4/17 Dr. Schur expresses wish to call for consultation Dr. Rigaud, famous radiologist, director of Curie Institute, Paris. Of course, agree readily, decision to await arrival. No change. Since hollow prosthesis is tapped and difficult to close, fluids enter and increase weight unnecessarily. Propose to prepare duplicate which could serve eventually also for insertion of radium.

4/20 From Paris advice against radium so long as malignancy of tumor uncertain. Therefore this plan abandoned and another consultation with Holzknecht arranged. H. insists on excision including surrounding, slightly modified Thiersch-surface.

4/23 Operation at Sanatorium Auersperg. Assistants: Berg, Weinmann, present Dr. Schur and Dr. Ruth Mack-Brunswick. ½ cc ephetonin, eucodal-scopolamine and locally 1%. Excision of Thiersch area in wide circumference of place with altered appearance including place where last papillae were excised, almost to bone of mandible but without removing periosteum. Afterward excision of greater part of scar-cord. Prosthesis inserted with cedenta under considerable pressure, Thiersch-graft of big flap from upper arm. Fairly severe bleeding from artery. Three ligatures. Effect of scopolamine good. Everything tolerated. Since patient moves mandible restlessly after operation, capistrum head bandage applied. Pneumovit injection. Advised Dr. Schur to try hormone treatment in view of favorable effect of vasoligature after first operation. Evening: Some drowsiness as during operation. Temporary confusion. Pulse good. Fluids can be drunk without difficulty.

4/26   Patient had 2 severe attacks of pain, otherwise feels much better, no fever. Capistrum unchanged. Histological report Erdheim. (No malignancy.)

9/8   During August, treated by Professor Kazanijan from Boston, partly in my consulting room. Prof. Kazanijan reduced and narrowed existing prosthesis considerably and finally made three prostheses. One of hard rubber, two with back part of soft rubber. These have doubtless the great advantage that they cannot lever at front teeth. Patient speaks much better with soft-rubber prosthesis but cannot smoke with it at all and bites his tongue. At right margin on tongue which has not recovered full sensitivity yet a suspect ulcer has developed. It decreased in size since this prosthesis has been used less, therefore excision abandoned.

1932/1/9   This time not better. Prosthesis 2 tried once again. Very uncomfortable but no pressure in precisely those places where pressure worst with prosthesis 3. Targesin. Some papillary hypertrophies at fold which protrudes right below.

1/27   Again swollen and worse. Also papilla seems more enlarged again after temporary diminution. Resection-prosthesis cannot be tolerated for more than ten minutes, therefore reduction of soft rubber not feasible.

3/7   Operation: $^{1}/_{2}$ cc modiscop and $^{3}/_{4}$% tutocaine locally. After local infiltration, posterior margin, otherwise visible in mirror only, is easily discernible; clear indication where to cut. Now cut around modified area of "mucous membrane" deep into healthy part with resulting extraction of wedge of ca. 1 cm thickness. Further, excision of remaining scar by scissors and attempt a suture. Successful only frontally. Attempt has to be abandoned below and above because of lack of movability and impossibility of undermining. Several sutures with silk and steel wire, packed with iodoform-gauze. Prosthesis fitted experimentally, insertion easy, removed again.

6/23   Increasing discomfort, not improved by rinsings. Investigation for sensitive places reveals one at buccal edge of residual antrum where epithelium lacks clear borders, appears somewhat modified and perhaps more papillary. Separated from this, close under the edge of antrum, two round white elevated papillomata, size of millet-seed, very sensitive to touch. Attempt at cauterization with Kerkhoff-paste causes immediate severe pain but leaves no special sensations.

7/18   Little discomfort until day before yesterday. Now speech disturbed again, sensations of swelling and tension. The two cauterized spots at orifice of antrum less sensitive. But swelling behind slope of existing velum still highly sensitive even though somewhat decreased. Some additional cauterization with Kerkhoff-paste. Immediate severe pain. Orthoform ointment.

7/29   Cauterized area and margin between soft palate, Thiersch-graft and nasal mucous membrane looks normal now. But there is a white place with the appearance of an hyperkeratous wart at the outer edge of the antrum within area of the antral mucous membrane, appr. size of hemp seed, sensitive to pressure. After psicoaine surface-anaesthesia and injection, painless destruction with diathermy (grade 4). In case procedure has to be repeated, still weaker current would be indicated.

8/10   In area where soft palate adjoins defect, a new granulating protuberance of pepper-corn size is to be seen. Discomfort, especially when speaking. This small area cauterized with Kerkhoff—otherwise with camillosan.

8/16 Another warty thickened overhanging edge at outer edge of antrum. Destroyed with diathermy (grade 3); coagulated piece scales off easily from hard base. Further, some superficial diathermy at nasal-palatal border.

10/4 Now somewhat larger area of 1.5:1 cm is sensitive with distinct papillary structure, the whole situated at outer and above all posterior area of residual antrum. Removal seems absolutely necessary.

10/6 After 1 allonal and 1 titran and after infiltration in palate, attempt at subbasal anaesthesia of ramus III. Excision of 2 cushions, at first under and inside residual antrum (piece No. 1) and then directly at inferior posterior edge including small piece of nasal mucous membrane. This includes removal of whole thickness of old scar. In second place some bone exposed with intention to remove clip. Base of processor pterygoideus. Intention not carried out since bone without doubt healthy. After this both places slightly diathermized and bridge between them cut with linear 3 mm broad diathermy cut to provide for scar from right to left. Third remaining red cushion at outer edge throughly destroyed with diathermy only. Some iodoform-gauze on bone in upper wound-hole, otherwise only orthoform and prosthesis.

11/10 Histological report Erdheim: Specially noticeable this time is widespread inflammation which covers the whole of the mucous membrane and is the consequence of excessive smoking. There is every evidence that the inflammation develops first and that the typical leukoplakia appears as its sequel. Further, both pieces contain places where the leukoplakia shows intensified proliferation of the epithelium, i. e. a precancerous stage; both pieces contain also places where stratifying globules begin to develop. But there is no serious growth into the depth; the underlying connective tissue is callous, scarred and enough has been removed to ensure the radical removal of the local proliferation of epithelium.

11/18 Patient has had very disagreeable severe influenza with otitis dextra with paracentesis, the latter surprisingly painless. Diathermy wounds healed with smooth scars. There is one slightly sensitive place at outer edge of residual antrum with minimal leukoplakia appearance; a second place far back below on protruding fold shows severe papillary modification, almost no sensitivity. Both places should be subjected to diathermy before long.

12/8 After infiltration surroundings of small tumor at palatinal arch delineated with diathermy-cuts, including adjacent piece of leukoplakia in downward direction. Further, cutting out of piece and coagulation of base, the latter restricted to area below warty thickening. Orthoform. Prescription: Perhydrol mouth wash to counteract tendency to formation of leukoplakia.

1933-2/15 Again complaints about "swellings," certain pressure when inserting prosthesis, etc. Rhinologist does not hold nasal catarrh responsible. Nothing to be seen apart from prosthesis being coated rather thickly with dried nasal secrete, partly encrusted which may cause pain. After swabbing one place with perhydrol, an evident leukoplakia shows distinct white discoloration. Swabbing repeated and patient instructed to resume the interrupted rinsings with hyperoxyd mouth wash. All frontal teeth painted with iod-iod-zinc. LR 3 filled provisionally.

4/6 "There has never been a worse week." Pressure, interference with speech. Nothing visible apart from some inflammation of nasal mucous membrane, no sensitiveness. This behind former ulcer area, corresponding to corner of prosthesis. Reduction there.

5/16 Patient complains of severe pain since yesterday. Place lingual right below appears swollen and irritated. Reduction of prosthesis there. Other place not sensitive but coagulated with diathermy after novocain injection. Orthoform, oxygen treatment of upper gum.

9/5 Diathermy of a strip where epithelium is thickened and very sensitive to pressure, from lingual surface across former scar-cord into overlaying groove. Further puncturing of single sensitive and thickly palpable point at outer edge of antrum. Orthoform.

9/15 Patient felt very ill subsequent to small operation, angina pectoris with coronary infarct.[e] Subsequent to this pneumonia of right lower lobe. All right again now.

1934/1/12 Pain, if anything, worse. No visible evidence except for greater tendency to bleed in sensitive place; probably once more beginning of papillary modification of surface epithelium. Since patient is not supposed to go out, attempt at superficial cauterization with Kerkhoff (original); causes violent pain; preliminary surface anaesthesia therefore preferable next time.

1/16 Worse; pain, pressure; insufficient relief with orthoform. At the point of last cauterization a wound with moderate sensitivity. The most painful spot further below on posterior declivity of fold which adjoins prosthesis outside. Small thickened place visible and palpable there since no compression at edge of prosthesis. Surface appears slightly papillary but same color as Thiersch-graft. Area painted with contralgin, prosthesis reduced there and lower part of modified surface cauterized with Kerkhoff; this time little pain. Probably again exactly same papilloma-formation as on former occasion.

[e]Actually "coronary insufficiency."

1/13 Consultation with Eisler[f] and Schur. Increasing pain. Both cauterized areas already much smaller, but still eroded and already flattened. Small wart on upper lip near corner of mouth, very hard and pointed, appearance of epithelioma incipiens, to be irradiated. Painful area to be irradicated with small doses in patient's home.

2/24 Patient has been irradiated by Eisler, feels no relief from pain. But last reduction of prosthesis, perhaps also retaining at night has improved pressure and lockjaw. Further reduction at highest convexity. In fold quite near lower edge of prosthesis new small area with papillary increase.

3/6 Pain said not to be better. Several sensitive places, especially above, area of normal mucous membrane covered with hard dry scraps of mucus and orthoform which are difficult to remove. The previously cauterized areas show irregular surface covering, in parts leukopl. white; only frontally below, where edge of prosthesis irritates scar-cord, distinct papillary raised area. Eisler suggests radium not x-ray for treatment of wart on lip.

[f]Radiologist.

3/10   Consultation with Fuhs,[g] Eisler, Schur. Decision to use old duplicate prosthesis for insertion of 50 mg radium at point of papillary proliferation. Cast of old prosthesis made, reduced in size.

3/23   50 mg radium inserted for 1 hour 12 min. All metal parts coated with lacquer and wax.

4/23   Insertion of 50 mg radium for 1 hour 12 min.

6/21   Check-up. Ulcer not healed, on the contrary bigger and more marked. Edge thickened papillary, especially mesial. Opening of mouth improved, perhaps through reduction of prosthesis. Pain not better. Prosthesis reduced further. Radium-prosthesis fitted.

6/27   Insertion of 50 mg radium for ½ hour avoiding direct contact. Condition to-day rather better than before. By agreement with Professor Fuhs to be repeated three to four times at intervals of several days.

7/6   Patient had epistaxis right side and violent attack of migraine preceded by scotoma, ascribed to radium. Probably wrongly, since bleeding originated in septum frontale. Advice: to carry out the four irradiations, to lengthen intervals, possibly slightly but not too much; if milder treatment decided on, to distribute the 100 mg planned for four sessions over five instead. Holder might profitably be shifted further forward by increasing cut-out place for it in prosthesis ca. 4 mm in forward direction.

7/30   Patient reacts each time with pain, swellings, tiredness and anginal attacks. Therefore decision to postpone another week.

[g] Radium specialist.

8/9   Had another very bad day: migraine, heart trouble, bad speech and severe local discomfort. Objectively: whole former swelling subsided and smooth. One spot, 3-4 mm diameter, discolored brown, probably consisting of papillae, distinctly sensitive to pressure, raised somewhat above surroundings. Perhaps residue of former, perhaps new papillary swelling. Otherwise whole mucous membrane much improved, smooth and clean. Prosthesis reduced slightly at the place. Wait and see!

8/30   Yesterday exceedingly bad day. To-day better. Place marked exactly on radium-prosthesis. Brown spot gone completely. Some reduction at edge.

9/24   Failure when trying to insert radium-prosthesis plus black guttapercha after generous reduction of clod. Prosthesis together with lower one is too big for mouth. Horizontal groove for holder is replaced by vertical one which, therefore, extends further upward and downward. This achieves additional distance of 3/4 cm and enlargement of field. 1 mm brass, all metal coated with wax. Recently very slight bleedings from mouth and nose. Wart on lower lip dropped off spontaneously. Dr. Schloss's[h] action based on conviction that radium with its minimal dosage of secondary importance, construction of new prosthesis of first importance. 50 mg radium for twenty-four minutes.

10/16   Papilloma vaguely visible but distinctly sensitive. Condition varies but lockjaw troublesome and pain and pressure persist. There seems no possibility for patient to come to my consulting room again. Another old prosthesis tried with guttapercha, still much too large, interferes with bite even without lower prosthesis which cannot be inserted. Insisted on further radium treatment against opposition.

11/16   50 mg radium inserted. This time much further backward than before since several distinct warty nodules have developed there whereas manifestations in old area have diminished further still. Radium should be applied soon again still further backward.

11/22   Check-up. Reaction said to be stronger than before. On day following treatment scintillating migraine as before and swellings. Old area looks all right but the two warty nodules prominent as before. Discussion with Dr. Schur: to try radium first, yet with awareness that diathermy would be preferable in this place. Advice to begin hormone treatment with androstin.

1935/3/20   General condition good but severe pressure-pain. Palpation shows sensitivity especially at edge of antrum and there mostly on area frontally outside, sharply circumscribed, of appr. 1 cm circumference, composed of very large coarse papillary groupings; this spot is fielded, circular, very slightly raised, slightly resistant and, of course, not movable on base of scar tissue. Conspicuous quality is its coarse spotting up to 1½ mm in diameter while all papillomata or warts till now were composed always of very small elements of quite equal size. This area is suspect and will have to be removed with diathermy unless it clears up spontaneously in the very near future. Patient not told yet. The two warts above the edge of prosthesis are definitely smaller though, perhaps more protruding, almost pedunculated but slightly hard.

3/23   Infiltration of area with 1½ cc novocaine without admixture of adrenalin and thorough coagulation of modified area; coagulated tissue lifted out of it with pincers. No manifestation of pain. Insufflation with orthoform and insertion of prosthesis after reduction of latter by 1-2 mm at this point.

h Radium specialist.

4/30   Electro-coagulation of both nodules probably including base and surroundings. Several small pieces scratched out with sharp spoon and preserved.

5/5   Patient had sudden violent pain when inserting prosthesis, therefore further reduction. Two places, one with the small papilloma-remnants mentioned before, the other higher above with dry brown slough adhering. The latter very hard to touch, only partly removable with hydrogen-hyperoxyd. Seems epithelium similar to black crusts of labial epithelioma.

5/6ⁱ   Patient reports great difficulty in inserting prosthesis. In the morning after cleaning insertion impossible. Yesterday still inserted with pain. To-day impossible, very upset, etc. Visit in consulting room. Apparent that rider right above slightly twisted which prevents prosthesis from slipping into place. An old nonfitting resection-prosthesis can be inserted. Imperfect insertion causes violent pain. Attempt to achieve insertion by reassurance, etc. fails. Decision to construct new prosthesis. Kerr-cast for new rider.

7/9   Two very bad days, then better after giving up ointment. Naturally, this has iSeventy-ninth birthday!

increased again the adherent slough. Cannot be removed fully with hydrogenhyperoxyd; probably has hyperkeratosis as base.

8/19   Eschar not removable, sharply bordered; slightly larger, more elevated, pressure on it probably responsible for discomfort. Keratosis almost certain. Tiny spot further backward, pin-point in size, shows similar condition. Formerly slough could be removed with care and patience, now tiny wart remains. Decision to electro-coagulate wart. In presence of Dr. Popper[j] injection 4% novocaine into base. ca. 1 cm^3 into three puncture-points. Cut around with diathermy needle. Puncture close to tumor. Lifted out with sharp spoon, proliferation of tumor into ca. 2-3 mm depth revealed. Circumference ca. 8-10 mm. Base coagulated, covered with phenol-camphora gauze, powdered with orthoform, prosthesis inserted. (1 cm^3 novocaine without adrenalin).

8/26   Report Erdheim:[k] "No cancer present but papillomata of this kind are precursors of cancer unless removed."

10/11   Excision of oviform papilloma, dark brown as before, with diathermy needle, excochleated, base coagulated. 4% novocaine without admixture.

1936/1/16 Operation: local injection of novocaine without adrenalin. Anaesthesis good except for one place backward above, then encircling by series of closely spaced diathermic needle punctures, then excochleation, and thorough fulguration of base.

2/11   Dr. Schur and Miss Anna complain of crusts, almost impossible to remove. In fact, rather small and not too many. If really not removable, cauterization with trichloracetic acid or superficial coagulation would be indicated. Scarlet-red ointment to be tried to relieve discomfort. At alveolar crest near UR 5 new white warty typical leukoplakia.

jSubstituting for Dr. Schur, who was vacationing.
kPathologist.

2/18   Crusts not worse thanks to plenty of eurecin ointment but not wholly removable. Probably based on samll dry keratoses, same as before last operation. Removal to be tried with trichloracetic acid. X-ray picture to be taken of leukoplakia in area of UR 5 to keep bone under observation. Instead of orthoform tentative painting with pantocaine, and eucerin ointment with admixture of 2% pantocaine to avoid possible irritating effect of orthoform.

2/20   Two places with brown crusts closely anterior to last operation defect cauterized with trichloracetic acid without visible white discoloration. Perhaps not enough. Upper leukoplakia at inner edge of antrum tested for pressure from prosthesis. Placed exactly where groove has been made in prosthesis to ease insertion. Not happy about it, should be removed some time.

7/13   Crusts reappeared. Trichloracetic acid in two places. Besides, there is now at posterior part of former leukoplakia on alveolar crest right above a circular ulcer bordered by kind of capsule; looks very suspicious since marginated circularly like node growing from depth. But node, as well as borders, not hard and hardly raised.

7/14   Submucous infiltration of described area at edge of alveolar crest backwards quite near to root of soft palate. 4% novocaine without adrenalin. Encircling into healthy tissue with diathermic needle punctures, then attempt to extirpate; violent pain relieved only by injection into node through wound. Probably corresponding to point near canalis sphenopalat. Then cutting out with knife and scissors since tissues not sufficiently softened by diathermy. Ad Erdheim. Then fulgurizing of borders and posterior part of focus. Anterior base is of smooth bone, not modified by disease.

7/16   Telephone message that examination shows epithelial carcinoma. (Report Erdheim.)

7/17   Examined slides with Erdheim in Jubilaeumsspital. They show carcinoma sharply bordered linearly by surrounding epithelium, itself, of course, strongly modified but not carcinomatous which forms overhanging wall; not extending far into depth and bordered underneath by scarred connective tissue. In other places of piece, not visible in present slides, carcinomatous tissue extended with some papillae into level of separating surface. Therefore decision to coagulate base only. For this purpose in Sanatorium Auersperg provision for nitrous oxide narcosis in case conduction-anaesthesia not successful.

7/18   Pantocaine after preceding thorough mouth cleaning and removal of brown crusts which come off easily now. Attempt at conduction-anaesthesia at foramen pterygoideum from outside. Not very successful. Isolation of formerly fulgurated soft tissue until bone exposed, then coagulation of base, with many interruptions because of pain. Then nitrous oxide narcosis, at first very successful, so that bone can be removed with Luer from edge of palate and also from medial wall of antrum. Further, very thorough fulguration of surroundings causing state of excitation and complaints of very violent pain. Afterward insertion of prosthesis and slight stuffing with iodoform gauze between prosthesis and operation area. Afterward coramine.

12/7   Daughter notices two small pits in lowest part of cheek which retain food remnants and are sensitive. Probably merely effect of shrinking. Above them hard nodule covered by mucous membrane. Higher above frontally small strongly protruding wart and frontally next to this flatter wart.

12/11   To-day small pit has unmistakable cancer appearance, walled margin. Diameter of infiltration hardly more than 6 mm. To be coagulated tomorrow. Strange that place which appeared unsuspicious on 12/7 leaves any doubt of the clinical diagnosis to-day.

12/12   Coagulation of ulcer. Novocaine injection with good effect in posterior part where tissue has loose appearance, less good frontally. Infiltration impossible above where bone lies immediately under mucous membrane, but unnecessary since anaesthesia has set in. First outer walls encircled with line of electric needle pricks, then piece of center excohleated, seems of non-suspicious consistency, finally base coagulated. Patient has no pain to start with; says towards end that he cannot stand any more, though I cannot think why. (!)

12/18 Lockjaw very disagreeable and apparently difficulty with swallowing; only fluids can be taken and cleaning is hardly possible. Short wave treatment, carried out as before in patient's home, gives some relief of pain and discomfort.

12/28 Some very bad days. After visit Dr. Berg orthoform-rods with effect of achieving wide opening of mouth so that prosthesis can be removed. Operation area bordered below by highly raised margin. Some hard keratoses which have caused pain.

1937/4/19 Dr. Schur has noticed for several days soft almost pedunculate movable wart grown from area of old pit after last operation. Macroscopic very suspicious appearance because of dentritic structure. Probably recurrence coming from depth after last operation. Decision to remove for examination, because of violent pain during last operation arrived at decision to do it in evipan-narcosis. If operation reveals that growth comes from depth, i. e. from bone, then ramus ascendens will have to be resected after microscopic examination.

4/22 Trial excision in evipan-narcosis. Cut around with needle, grasped with hooklet and separated from base partly with knife since it resists loosening with sharp spoon. Base of wound consists of hard connective tissue, no softer place where spoon can enter, as anticipated. Surroundings and base electro-coagulated and insufflated with orthoform. No bandage. Upper prosthesis inserted, patient to insert lower one after waking up. Specimen to Chiari.[1]

1938/1/17 Lockjaw, if anything, worse. Suspicious place rather more convex. Inflammation of surroundings receded. Observe some more days.

1/22 Operation Sanatorium Auersperg. After some difficulties a handle for the diathermy apparatus has been found, long enough to reach tumor form left. Evipan. Encircling of piece of tumor with diathermy needle. Failure to secure it with sharp spoon since tissue hard, scarred, adheres tightly to base. No instrument present for cutting at base, squeezing out of pulpy masses. After excision with scissors (ad Chiari), diathermy coagulation of this place and all other modified areas; thoroughly, but smallness of burner which had to be used leaves doubt whether everywhere. Both warts destroyed by needle. Then atheroma in left submandibular area encircled and cut out with scissors without causing injury. Complete suture after one ligature. Orthoform powder on mouth wound. Prosthesis, which broke shortly before operation, repaired meanwhile, inserted. Lower prosthesis reduced slightly to ease removal and insertion.

[1] Pathologist.

2/19 Excision of suspect wart in area of last operation. (Histologically negative.)

6/2 Last examination before departure to England. Keratosis in one place, in form of recurrent brown crust. Several places not quite all right but not suspicious according to previous experience.

9/7 Examination in London. Dr. Exner had been ready to remove quick-growing cancer anteriorly to last operation site, in area of protruding skin-fold which had developed into unmistakable tumor, when he and Dr. Schur noticed second very suspicious place behind and over last operation-site, near to passage into maxilla. This place definitely sensitive to pressure and immovable towards ramus ascendens as ascertained in examination immediately after journey to London. Therefore decision to operate tomorrow and, if necessary, to exarticulate upper part of ramus ascendens, so as to remove suspicious bone and danger of increasing lockjaw.

9/8 Operation by Prof. Pichler, at London Clinic. Narcosis first evipan, continued with nitrogenoxydul via nasal tube. Lip divided and cut continued along nose to enable good access for once. Then excision of cheek tumor with diathermy needle and, finally, of wholly modified tissue backward above over anterior edge of ramus ascendens. Excision of large pieces of very hard tough tissue. Macroscopically no appearance of cancer but of callous scar. Removed until needle meets soft healthy muscle, though perhaps not everywhere reliably in modified tissue. Finally, fixed anterior edge of ramus ascendens is exposed and coagulated to extent of 1½ cm. When impression gained that everything removed, prosthesis inserted, wound cavity insufflated with orthoform, and tamponed with 5% iodoform-gauze.

9/17 Report on excision from cheek: no definite cancer, microscopically precancerous stage. Posterior pieces so far not examined owing to some error.

1939/2/11 Dr. Schur reports that end of December a fairly large sequestrum was discharged followed by temporary improvement. Then again pain and a node and ulcer which Schur considers carcinomatous. Since patient cannot be subjected to another operation, radium seems indicated. Asks for report on previous dosage.

2/15 Advice to coagulate additional to radium. Report on doses applied earlier.

2/20 Dr. Schur reports on impending visits by Drs. Trotter and Lacassagne, the latter to give the radium treatment in Paris; asks whether I would come to Paris, if necessary. Answer: slides sent and ready to come but do not think necessary since coagulation can be done in Paris.

2/28 Letter Dr. Schur: x-ray negative, biopsy suspect (Dr. Exner), examination by Drs. Trotter and Lacassagne from Paris. Dr Trotter wants to wait further week. Dr. Lacassagne wants another surgical opinion in case of another biopsy.

5/15 Exner: recurrence high above in antrum. Operation not indicated any more. Radium has been applied by way of prosthesis for two hours daily, no ill effects, no headaches; additional to this deep x-ray irradiations. Tumor receded but metastases.

5/29/46 Letter Dr. Exner: Further applications of radium in small doses, two hours daily, besides deep x-ray irradiations. Metastases and extension of disease into eye-socket. Death on 9/23/39 after being unconscious for twenty-four hours.

CONTRIBUTORS

Lieutenant Colonel Madelaine A. Bader, Army Nurse Corps, Walter Reed Army Institute of Nursing, Washington, D.C.

Dr. Harry L. Berman, Department of Radiation Therapy, Sinai Hospital of Baltimore, Baltimore, Maryland

Dr. Thomas J. Bridges, Jr., Associate Attending Neurological Surgeon, Neurological Institute, Columbia-Presbyterian Medical Center, New York, New York

Dr. Arthur C. Carr, Professor (Medical Psychology), Department of Psychiatry, College of Physicians and Surgeons, Columbia University, New York, New York, Chairman, Professional Advisory Board, Foundation of Thanatology

Dr. S. Gordon Castigliano, Chief, Head and Neck Service, American Oncological Hospital, Philadelphia, Pennsylvania

Evelyn F. Cooper, Director, Social Service Department, Memorial Hospital for Cancer and Allied Diseases, New York, New York

Alice Costello, R.N., Head and Neck Service, Memorial Hospital for Cancer and Allied Diseases, New York, New York

Dr. Fred F. Cowan, Chairman, Department of Pharmacology, University of Oregon Dental School, Portland, Oregon

Dr. Alben Curtis, St. Jude Children's Research Hospital, Memphis, Tennessee

Dr. Clifton O. Dummett, Assistant Dean, School of Dentistry, University of Southern California, Los Angeles, California; Past President, International Association for Dental Research

Elaine A. Finnberg, Foundation of Thanatology, New York, New York

Dr. Ivan K. Goldberg, Associate, Department of Psychiatry, College of Physicians and Surgeons, Columbia University, New York, New York

Dr. Harvey Gralnick, School of Dental and Oral Surgery, Columbia University, New York, New York

Georgia Hall, R.D.H., Coordinator of Dental Services, A. Holly Patterson Home for the Aged, Uniondale, New York

Dr. Ian W. D. Henderson, Department of Pharmacology, Faculty of Medicine, University of Ottawa, Ontario, Canada

Dr. Frederic P. Herter, Professor of Surgery, College of Physicians and Surgeons, Columbia University, New York, New York

Dr. Alfred S. Ketcham, Chief of Surgery and Director of Clinics, National Cancer Institute, National Institutes of Health, Bethesda, Maryland

Dr. Austin H. Kutscher, Associate Professor and Director, New York State Psychiatric Institute, School of Dental and Oral Surgery, Columbia University, New York, New York; President, Foundation of Thanatology

Harlan A. Kutscher, Student, College of Physicians and Surgeons, Columbia University, New York, New York

Lillian G. Kutscher, Foundation of Thanatology, New York, New York

Constance Lamb, Supervisor of Social Work, Department of Surgery, The Presbyterian Hospital in the City of New York, Columbia-Presbyterian Medical Center, New York, New York

Dr. Martin I. Lorin, Assistant Attending Pediatrician, Babies Hospital, The Presbyterian Hospital in the City of New York, Columbia-Presbyterian Medical Center, New York, New York

Dr. Susan Mellette, Assistant Professor of Medicine, Cancer Chemotherapy, Virginia Commonwealth University, Medical College of Virginia, Richmond, Virginia

Dr. Edward H. Montgomery, Assistant Professor of Pharmacology, University of Oregon Dental School, Portland, Oregon

Dr. Manuel Ochoa, Jr., Associate Attending Physician, Memorial Hospital for Cancer and Allied Diseases, New York, New York

Dr. David Peretz, Associate, Department of Psychiatry, College of Physicians and Surgeons, Columbia University, New York, New York; Chairman, Research Committee, Foundation of Thanatology

Helen Pettit, Professor of Nursing, Department of Nursing, College of Physicians and Surgeons, Columbia University, New York, New York

Elizabeth R. Prichard, Assistant Professor, Department of Medicine (Medical Social Service), College of Physicians and Surgeons, Columbia University, New York, New York

Dr. M. B. Quigley, Oral Physiology Research Laboratory, Veterans Administration Hospital, Houston, Texas

Rev. Robert B. Reeves, Jr., Chaplain, The Presbyterian Hospital in the City of New York, Columbia-Presbyterian Medical Center, New York, New York

Dr. Norman G. Schaaf, Chief, Dental and Maxillofacial Prosthetic Services, Roswell Park Memorial Institute, Buffalo, New York

Dr. Paul Scheman Director of Dentistry, Kingsbrook Jewish Medical Center, Brooklyn, New York

Dr. Bernard Schoenberg, Associate Clinical Professor, Department of Psychiatry, College of Physicians and Surgeons and Associate Dean, College of Physicians and Surgeons, Columbia University, New York, New York; Chairman of the Executive Committee of the Foundation of Thanatology

Dr. I. L. Shannon, Director, Oral Physiology Research Laboratory, Veterans Administration Hospital, and The University of Texas Dental Branch, Houston, Texas

INDEX

Elaine A. Finnberg

A. Holly Patterson Home for the Aged, 185
Abandonment, of the dying patient, 11; *see also* Isolation
Acetylcysteine, 160
Actinomycin D, 108
Adaptive mechanisms: use by oral cancer patient, 53-56; use by patient's family, 57-58
Addiction, drug: of oral cancer patient, 30; physician response to, 147
Adolescent, 156
Adrenal steroids, and treatment of bacterial infection, 84
Adrenolytic agents, 120
Alcaroid, 40
Alcohol ingestion, and the dying patient, 45, 79
Alevaire, 40
Alimentary tract decompression, 90
American Cancer Society, 32, 225
Amethopterin, 160
Amigen, 79
Aminopyrine, and association with leukopenia, 89
Ampicillin, and treatment of infection in oral cancer patient, 85
Anabolic agents, 82
Anabolism, 78
Analgesic agents: and association with leukopenia, 89; and control of oral cancer pain, 86, 87; narcotic, use of, 143-149; non-narcotic, use of, 143-149; *see also* specific agents
Androgen therapy, 82
Anemia, in dying patient, 78, 81
Anesthetics, topical, in control of oral cancer pain, 86; *see also* Xylocaine
Anger: of bereaved, 226; of staff, 203
Angular stomatitis, 29

Anorexia nervosa, 156
Anosmia, 37
Anoxia, caused by cardio-pulmonary disturbances, 90
Antianxiety agents: use of in care of oral cancer patient, 143-145; use of in care of terminally ill patient, 143-145; use of in control of oral cancer pain, 86
Antibiotic therapy: and control of oral cancer pain, 86; and oral cancer patient, 84-85; and surgery, 84
Anticancer drugs, side effects of, 159; *see also* Antitumor agents; Chemotherapy, cancer
Anticholinergic agents, 82, 118
Antidepressant agents, 46, 128-130; use of in care of oral cancer patient, 147; use of in care of terminally ill patient, 147; use of in control of oral cancer pain, 86; *see also* Monoamineoxidase inhibitor antidepressants; Tricyclic antidepressants
Antiemetic agents, 116-117; *see also* Phenothiazine derivatives
Antimicrobial agents, in control of oral cancer pain, 86
Antipsychotic agents, 116-117; use of in care of oral cancer patient, 143-145; use of in care of terminally ill patient, 143-145; use of in control of oral cancer pain, 86; *see also* Phenothiazine derivatives
Antipyretic drugs, use in controlling fever, 85
Antisialagogues, 164
Antitumor agents: alkylating agents, 107; antimetabolites, 108; antitumor antibiotic, 108; hormones, 108; mechanism of action, 106-108; plant alkaloids, 108

Anxiety: of dying patient, 77; as family reaction to fatal illness, 58; and response to pain, 85
Anxiolytic sedative agents, 122-128; drug interactions, 135; indications for, 122; pharmacological effects of, 122; see also Benzodiazepine derivatives; Carbamate derivatives; "Minor tranquilizers"
Apathy, of dying patient, 77
APC, in control of oral cancer pain, 86
Arabinosylcytosine, 108
Ascorbic acid, 78, 81
Aspirator, mechanical, use of in oral hygiene, 169
Aspirin, 36; antipyretic effect of, 146; in control of oral cancer pain, 86, 87
Asthma, and grief reaction, 68-69
Astringents, in control of oral cancer pain, 86
Atelectasis, 90
Atropine and derivatives, 164
Attitudes toward death: of dying patient, 216; in modern society, 214, 224, 225
Avitaminosis, 88
Azotemia, in dying patient, 78
Bader, Madelaine A., 195-207
Banthine, 164
Barbiturates: and association with leukopenia, 89; in control of oral cancer pain, 86
Bedridden patient, dental care of, 168
Benzocaine lozenges and paste, 37, 86
Benzodiazepine derivatives, 126-128; drug interactions of, 128; mechanisms of action, 126; pharmacological effects of, 126; side effects of, 127-128; therapeutic uses of, 127
Bereaved, the: reaction of, 226; role of dentist in working with, 77-73
Bereavement: grief reactions in, 68, 71-73; and identification with lost loved object, 72; oral involvement in, 69, 71-73; and psychological disturbances, 71-72; and somatic disturbances, 68-69, 71-72; and role of social worker, 225-226
Berman, Harry L., 92-98
Biopsy, as cause of infection, 83
Body-image: alteration caused by cancer surgery, 59; of dying child, 160, 228-232; see also Disfigurement; Self-image
Body resistance to infection, 83
Bone marrow depression, 119
Breast cancer, effectiveness of chemotherapy in, 109
Bridges, Thomas J., Jr., 99-105
Bronchial asthma, 135
Bruxism, in bereabement, 71
Burkitt's lymphoma, effectiveness of chemotherapy in, 109
Burning mouth syndrome, and grief reaction, 68-69
Burning tongue, and grief, 68-69
Butyrephenone derivatives, 121-122; see also Phenothiazine derivatives
Cachexia: as cause of anemia, 89; as cause of leukopenia, 89; in dying patient, 77
Caffeine, 37
Calorie intake, of dying patient, 79
Cancer: and grief reaction, 68-69; individual susceptibility variations, 57; meaning of in modern society, 57; prognosis, 31, 33, 47; therapy of, 108-111; see also Antitumor agents; Chemotherapy, cancer; Oral Cancer
Cancer, in child, see Child, terminally ill
Candidiasis, 83, 150
Carbamate, 123
Carbamate derivatives, 123-126; see also Meprobamate
Cardio-pulmonary disturbances, in dying patient, 90
Care, see Oral care; Patient; Terminal.

Caries: in dying patient, 77; prevention of, 82, 86, 170
Carisoprodol, 123
Carotid body syndrome, 43
Carr, Arthur C., 3-15
Castigliano, S. Gordon, 31-51
Chaplin, *see* Pastor; Pastoral care
Chemotherapy, cancer, 106-111; attitude of physician toward, 106; complications of, 86, 88, 89, 154; effect on cancer cells, 106-107; effect on normal cells, 106-107; effectiveness of, 108-109; recovery from, 78; and side effects of, 53, 109-111; use of, 90
Child, dying: body-image of 60; and care of mouth, 157-161; and elective procedures, 158; and oral care during disease remission, 165-166; and oral gratification, 157; and oral problems of, 157-161; and role of dentist, 158, 165-166
Child, as patient, psychological management of, 6
Child, terminally ill, 150-155; management of, 151-155; psychological aspects of, 151; rejection of, 152, 55; *see also* Oral care, in terminally ill child
Chloramphenicol, as cause of thrombocytopenia, 89
Chloraseptic spray, use of in control of pain in oral cancer, 86
Chlordiazepoxide, 126, 128
Chlorphenesin, 123
Chlorpromazine, 60, 90, 113, 114, 115, 116, 118, 119, 129; *see also* Phenothiazine derivatives, Thorazine
Choriocarcinoma, 111
Chorioepithelioma, and effectiveness of chemotherapy in, 109
Cingulotomy, and control of intractable pain in oral cancer, 87
Circumoral dermatitis, 29
Cleft palate, 161
Clorpactic solution irrigation, 37

Codeine, 36, 145, 146; use of in control of pain in oral cancer, 86, 87
Colitis, ulcerative, and grief reaction, 68-69
Colon cancer, 107
Comatose patient, oral care of, 99
Communication: as byproduct of good oral care, 211; between dentist and parents, 151; between dentist and physician, 155, 158; by dying patient, 20-21; between family and health professional, 181; among health professionals, viii, 158; importance of mouth in, 20-21; importance of oral care in, 20-21; methods available of, 211; and need for honesty between child patient and dentist, 181; between patient and staff, 56, 64; between physician and patient, 25, 55, 92-93; problems after oral cancer surgery, 53
Community dentistry, 181-182
Community resources: lack of for terminally ill patient, 224-225, *see also* Terminally ill patient, care facilities for; for prosthodontic care, -175
Compazine, 145
Congestive heart failure, 90
Constipation, 45, 81
Conversion reaction, hysterical or atypical facial pain in bereavement, 71
Cooper, Evelyn F., 208-213
Corticosteroid creams, 43
Corticosteroids, 49; side effects of, 159; topical application in control of oral cancer pain, 86-87
Cortisone, in care of oral cancer patient, 164
Cosmesis, *see* Disfigurement
Cosmetic deformity, *see* Disfigurement
Costello, Alice, 190-194
Covicone cream, 43

Cowan, Fred F., 112-142
Cranial nerve sectioning, and control of pain, 30, 87
Cryosurgery, 27
Curtis, Alban B., 150-155
Cyclophosphamide, 107
Cystic fibrosis, oral treatment in, 160
Cytopenia, as side effect of cancer chemotherapy, 109
Dakin's solution irrigation, 37
Darvon, 36, 86, 145, 146
Death: changes in our societal attitudes toward, 7; as defeat, 9, 18; denial, of medical student, 18; with dignity, 8, 48-49, 62, 196; fear of, see Fear, of death; as an ongoing process, 31; as taboo topic in our society, 7
Death, impending: and oral disease, 114; and psychosomatic pain, 114
Decubiti, and effect on oral tissues, 91
Dehydration, in dying patient, 78
Delusions about mouth, and bereavement, 71
Demerol, 37, 145, 146, 147; see also meperidine
Denial: as adaptive mechanism to cope with loss, 71; by patient of fatal prognosis, 64-66, 232
Dental care, of terminally ill patient: of bedridden patient, 168; and and effect on family, 167; and effect on health personnel, 167; financial problems, 222; of hospitalized patient, 169; of nursing home patient, 169; of patient at home, 169; procedures in, 167-170; and psychological state of patient, 168; societal attitudes toward, 209; see also Oral care; Oral hygiene
Dental extractions, as cause of infection, 83
Dental history of bereaved, as a part of oral care, 72-73

Dental hygienist, role of in care of geriatric patient, 188
Dentist: and community dentistry, 181-182; and drug therapy, 114-115, 119, 128, 130; and oral side effects of cancer chemotherapy, 109-111; as part of the medical team, 2, 4, 17-23, 184; and procedures in care of dying patient, 163-164, 165-166; and responsibility for care of dying patient, 162-166; role of in care of the bereaved, 71-73; role of in care of dying patient, 17-23, 29, 46, 47-48, 112, 162-166, 178-183; and treatment of oral cancer patient, 163-164
Dentist, in care of terminally ill child: management of terminally ill child, 151-155; psychological aspects of care, 151-152; role of in care of terminally ill child, 154-155, 158, 165-166; working with parents, 151
Dentistry: community, 181-182; and the dying patient, 162-166, 212-213; modern concept of, 178-179; restorative, 180
Dentures, 185; cleaning of, 169; use by terminally ill patient, 163, 168
Deoxyuridylic acid, 108
Dependence, of patient on physician, 62
Dependence, of terminally ill, 11
Depression: in bereavement, 71; as family reaction to fatal illness, 58; of oral cancer patient, 232; and response to pain in dying patient, 85
Detachment, of dying patient, 77
Diabetes mellitus, and grief reaction, 68-69
Diagnosis, fatal: stages of emotional reaction to diagnosis, 56; whether or not to tell patient, 55, 92-93; see also Communication
Diarrhea, 81

Diazepam, 114, 126
Dietary and nutritional problems, of dying patient, 77-79; anorexia, 77; azotemia, 78; cachexia, 77; causes of, 88; as complications of treatment, 77; dehydration, 78; feeding, 79; length of time of patient restriction to diet, 80; malnutrition, 77; physical impediment to passage of food, 78; psychological problems, 81; weight loss, 77
Dietary therapy, in dying patient, 78-82; calcium, 78; carbohydrates, 78; iron, 81; magnesium, 78; potassium, 78; protein, 78; roughage, 80; vitamin supplementation, 86; vitamins, 78
Diets, use of by dying patient, 79-82; liquid, 79; soft, 79-81; supplementation, 5-6, 81-82
Dilaudid, 37
Disease, see Oral disease
kopenia, 89
Disfigurement, 180-181; caused by surgery, 52, 143; see also Body-image; Self-image
Disfigurement, of dying patient, 104; caused by surgery, 231; coping with, 223-224; management of, 27; see also Body-image; Self-image
Diuretics, 120
DNA depolymerization, 108; synthesis, 107
Dornavac, see Pancreatic nuclease
Drooling, 42, 86; control of, 28-29; control of in oral cancer patient, 164
Drug therapy, complications of, 186, 187
Dulcolax, 82
Dummett, Clifton O., 178-183
Dying, with dignity, ix; fear of, see Fear, of dying
Dying child, see Child, dying
Dying's dignity, 143

Dying patient: cardiopulmonary disturbances of, 90; care of by radiotherapist, 92-98; classification of, 46-48; dietary and nutritional problems of, 77-79; dietary therapy of, 78-82; drug therapy of, 112, 134; family reactions, 24, 27; and fear of dying, 164-165; final days of life, 49-50; gastrointestinal disturbances of, 90; hematologic complications, of 88-90; and home care, 32; hospitalization of, 32; need for programs to provide oral care to, 212; and nursing homes, 32; nutritional maintenance of, 27-28; oral care to, 212; oral care of, 31, 33-51, 77, 83, 91; and oral hygiene, 77, 85, 91; and oral infection, 82-85; oral manifestations of systemic disease, 77; and pain, 85-87; and participation in care, 217-220; role of physician in caring for, 24-30; therapy of, 78, 79, 84-85; and transfer from hospital, 224; treatment goals for, 32; voluntary euthanasia, 49; see also Health professionals; Oral care, of dying patient; Oral care, of terminally ill patient; Social workers; Terminal patient; Terminally ill patient
Dying patient, elderly, 164-165
Dyspnea, 90
Dysproteinemia, 84, 88
Dystonic syndrone, 119
Eczematoid dermatitis, 43
Education, dental, in oral care of dying patient, 17, 19, 21-23; and patient priority, 18
Education, medical, in oral care of dying patient, 22
Education, medical, dental and nursing: lack of training in care of terminally ill and bereaved, 7-8; lack of training in oral cancer patient care

Education, of medical team to work with dying patient and bereaved, 202-206; benefits of for staff, 203
Elective procedures, in children, 158
Emotional response, of health professionals to dying patient, 155
Endoscopy, as cause of oral infection, 83
Epinephrine, 117-118
Erythrocyte formation, in dying patient, 78
Escape, as family reaction to fatal illness, 58
Euthanasia, voluntary, 49
Family, the: and acceptance of oral cancer surgery, 193-194; and bereavement, 225-226; and community dentistry, 182; and home care of terminally ill patient, 224-225; reactions to cosmetic disfigurement of dying patient, 27; reactions to failure of cancer treatment of dying patient, 24; role of in care of oral cancer patient, 193-194; role of nurse in helping, 201
Fear, of death, by family, 8; by physicians, 8-9
Fear, of dental procedures, and perception of dentist, 70-71; and psychological implications of, 70
Fear, of dying, and effect on dental care, 164-165
Feeding, of dying patient, 79, 103-104
Ferrous sulfate, 81
Fever, in dying patient, 78, 85; control of, 85
5-fluorouracil, 108
Finnberg, Elaine,
Freud, Sigmund, as oral cancer patient, 3-6, 235-253; case extract, 235-253; and psychological aspects of oral cancer, 3-6
Funeral practices, 13
Gamma globulin injections, for treatment of oral infection, 84
Gastrointestinal cancer, 107; and effectiveness of chemotherapy in, 109

Gastrointestinal disturbances, in dying patient, 90
Gentian violet, 38, 164; use of in children, 160
Geriatric death, see Dying patient, elderly
Geriatric dental care, 184-189; as affected by existing disease conditions, 185-186, 188; in nursing homes, 184-189; oral complications of drug therapy, 186; problems caused by denture wearing, 185
Gingival necrosis, 165
Gingival resorption, 169
Gingivitis, 150; ulcerative, 160
Glucocorticoid, in treatment of bacterial infection, 84
Glucose-6-phosphate dehydrogenase deficiency, 88
Goldberg, Ivan K., 143-149
Gralnick, Harvey, 143-149
Gram-negative infections, and leukopenia, 89
Grief and mourning, see Bereavement
Guilt, of parents when child has fatal illness, 57
Hall, Georgia, 184-189
Head and neck cancer, oral care of, 94-95; see also Oral Cancer
Head and neck cancer surgery, see Postoperative nursing, oral cancer care
Health professionals: and avoidance of death, 9; and emotional response to dying patient, 155; and goal of cure, 9; role of in care of dying child, 157; role of in care of terminal patient, vii; role of interdisciplinary team in care of dying patient, 224
Hematologic complications, in dying patient, 88-90; anemia, 88-89; leukopenia, 89; thrombocytopenia, 89-90
Hemoglobinopathy, 88
Hemorrhage, 43-44

Index

Henderson, Ian W. D., 52-67
"Heroic measures," 7-8, 18
Herter, Frederic P., vii
Hodgkin's disease, and effectiveness of chemotherapy in, 109
Home care, of dying patient, 32
Hospice, and management of dying patient, 8
Hospital: function of defined, 178; oral care in, 179; transfer from and effect on family and patient, 224
Hospitalization, of dying patient, 178
Hygiene, see Oral hygiene
Hydrogen peroxide irrigation, 37, 41
Hyoscine, 37
Hypersensitivity reaction, as Phenothiazine derivatives side effect, 119
Hypnosis, in pain management of dying patient, 37
Hypochondriasis and bereavement, 72
Hypoglobulinemia, 84
Hypoproteinemia, 78
Hypoprothrombinemia, 88
Hypotension: arterial, 117; postural, 117
Hypothyroid disease, 135
Hypotonic solutions, in care of oral cancer patient, 164
Illness, as threat, 215
Immunoglobulins, in dying patient, 83
"Incurable patient, the": control of pain in, 65; psychological management of emotional needs of, 62-67; psychological reactions of patient and family, 61-65; reaction of hospital staff to, 62; reaction of nurses to, 63; reaction of physicians to, 63; role of staff in psychological caring for, 64-67; see also Terminally ill patient
Infection: control of, 29; in oral cancer patient, 38; susceptibility to in patients receiving antitumor agents i.e., cancer chemotherapy), 111; see also Oral infection
Insomnia, and effect on oral tissues, 90
Intellectualization, as adaptive mechanism to cope with loss, 71
Intensive care unit, 182
"Interpersonal relationships," as technique in care of dying patient, 196
Intrahepatic obstructive jaundice, 119
Intra-oral cancer, see Oral cancer
Intravenous alcohol, 37
Intubation, decompressive, in treatment of gastrointestinal disturbances, 90
Isocarboxazid, 130
Isolation: of bereaved, 226; coping with in dying patient, 224; of dying child, 160; of oral cancer patient, 231-232; see also Abandonment, Self-image
Isuprel, 40
Karo syrup irrigation, 40
Kenalog, in Orabase, 86-87
Ketcham, Alfred S., 24-30
Kidney disease, chronic, oral treatment in, 160-161
Kordremul, 45
Kutscher, Austin H., 16-23, 143-149
Kutscher, Harlan A., 143-149
Kutscher, Lillian G.
Lamb, Constance, 214-227
Largactil, use of in postoperative patient, 60
Laryngopharynx cancer, 26-30
Leukemia, 89, 152-153, 165; and effectiveness of chemotherapy, in 109; oral treatment in, 160
Leukoerythroblastosis, 88
Leukopenia, 83, 119
Librium, 147; use of in control of pain in oral cancer, 86; see also Chlordiazepoxide
Life, prolongation of, 85
Life expectancy, of dying patient, and oral care, 163, 165

Lobotomy, prefrontal, 37; and control of intractable pain in oral cancer, 87
Local anesthetics, *see*: Anesthetics, topical; Xylocaine
Loneliness, and effect on oral tissues, 91
Lorin, Martin I., 156-161
Loss: death as one of the crises involving loss, 202; and role in pathogenesis of oral disorders, 71-72; and significance of mouth, 69-73; and use of adaptive mechanisms, 70
Lung cancer, and effectiveness of chemotherapy in, 109
Lung emphysema, 135
Lymph nodes, in oral cancer, 83
Lymphocytic leukemia, 150
Lymphoid malignancy, 88
Lymphoma, 89; and effectiveness of chemotherapy in, 109
Lymphosarcoma, 107
Maalox, 41
"Major tranquilizers," 122
Malaise, 81
Malnutrition, in dying patient, 77
Maltsupex, 45
Marplan, 46; *see also* Isocarboxazid
Matulane, *see* Methylhydrazine
Maxillectomy, radical, 193
Maxillofacial prosthesis, use of with dying patient, 173-175
Mebutamate, 123
Medical help seeking, 55
Medical personnel, *see* Health professionals
Medical student, attitudes toward death, 18
Medical team: and acceptance of dentist as member, 17, 22; and communication between dental staff and medical staff, 22; and communication between nurse and dental hygienist, 22; education of to work with dying patient and

bereaved, 9, 202-206; *see also* Project CAM
Medicine, technological advances in, 52; altering "terminal" aspects of many diseases, 16; causing moral, ethical and social issues because of ability to prolong life indefinitely, 7
Melanoma, and effectiveness of chemotherapy in, 109
Mellette, Susan, 106-111
Membranes of skin or mucous, erosion of, 83
Meperidine, 120, 135; *see also* Demerol
Meprobamate, 123-126, 127; as cause of thrombocytopenia, 89; drug interactions, 125-126; pharmacological effects of, 123, 126; therapeutic uses of, 124
6-mercaptopurine, 108
"Mercy killing," 49
Metamucil, 45
Methadone, 146
Methotrexate, 108, 110, 165; and effect on oral tissues, 165; *see also* Amethopterin
Methyl prednisolone, 84
Methylhydrazine, 108
Milk of Magnesia, 45
Miltown, use of in control of pain in oral cancer, 86
Mineral oil, 45
"Minor tranquilizers," 122, 123, 125, 126
Moniliasis, 86; *see also* Oral moniliasis
Monoamine-oxidase inhibitor antidepressants, 130-132; drug interaction, 131, 135; pharmacological effects of, 128, 129, 130-131; side effects of, 130-131; therapeutic use of, 128, 129
Monoamine-oxidase inhibitors, 46
Montgomery, Edward H., 112-142
Morphine, 37, 145, 146, 147, 148; drug interaction, 135; pharmaco-

logical effects of, 134; side effects of, 134
Mouth: care of in dying child, 157-161; and oral stimulation, 157; psychological significance of, 69-70, 156-157; and self-gratification, 157; as site of early losses, 69-70; symbolic significance of, 12-13; symbolic significance of and regression, 12
Mouth wash, use of by terminal patient, 163, 164
Mucomyst, 40; see also Acetylcysteine
Mucositis, 82
Multiple myeloma, and effectiveness of chemotherapy in, 109
Muscular tension, in bereavement, 71
Mycolog ointment, 43
Mycostatin, 38; see also Nystatin
Myelophthisic anemia, 88
Narcotic agents, use of in dying patient, 79
Narcotic analgesics, see Morphine
Nardil, 46; see also Phenelzine
Nasal feeding, of dying patient, 79
National Institutes of Health, clinical cancer training programs of, 19
Nausea, caused by gastrointestinal disturbance, 90
Necrosis, in oral cancer patient, 83
Neo-Cortef cream, 43
Neuroblastoma, oral complications of, 160
Neuroleptic agents: drug interaction, 135; indications for, 115; see also Antidepressants; Anxiolytic sedatives; Butyrophenone derivatives; Phenothiazine derivatives; Thioxanthene derivatives
Neurotic and psychotic mechanisms, in bereavement, 72
Neurotoxicity, as side effect of cancer chemotherapy, 110
Neutropenia, 84; and predisposition to infection, 89
Nialamide, 130

Niamid, 46; see also Nialamide
Nilevar, see Norethandrolone
Nitrogen mustard, 107
Norethandrolone, 82
Normocytic anemia, 89
Nupercaine lozenges, 37; use of in control of pain in oral cancer, 86
Nurse, role of in care of dying patient, 195-207; and attitudes toward death, 196; and interpersonal relationship techniques for care of dying patient, 196; and working with family of patient, 200-201; and working with medical team, 198-206
Nurse, role of in caring for oral cancer patient, 56; and postoperative management of patient, 190-194; and psychosocial care of family, 193-194; and psychosocial care of patient, 193
Nursing homes, need for dental services, 188; see also A. Holly Patterson Home for the Aged
Nursing services, and home care of terminally ill patient, 225
Nursing staff, role of in care of geriatric patient, 188
Nutrition, of dying patient, 44-45
Nutritional maintenance, and terminal patient, 27-28; feeding methods of, 28
Nystatin, 160, 161
Obesity, and grief reaction, 68-69
Ochoa, Manuel, Jr., 77-91
Odor, mouth, control of, 29
Odor, in oral cancer patient, 37-38; control of, 164
Opiates, 36
Orahesive bandage, and control of pain in oral cancer, 86
Oral cancer: coping with patient reactions, 53-57; coping with psychological fears involved, 53; metastasis and management of patient, 26-27; morbidity, 186; nutritional maintenance in, 27-28; oral hy-

giene in, 28-30; surgery in, 52; susceptibility to, 186; to tell or not to tell the patient, 25; therapy in, 25-26; therapy in geriatric patient with, 184-189; and treatment by dentist, 163-164; use of analgesics in, 143-149; use of psychopharmacological agents in, 143-149

Oral cancer, complications of: disfigurement, 27; drooling, 28-29; infection, 29; mouth odor, 29; nutritional maintenance, 27-28; oral hygiene, 28-30; pain, 29-30

Oral cancer patient, the: psychological effect of enforced dependence, 9; vs. self-care, 11

Oral care: in chronic renal disease, 160-161; in cystic fibrosis, 160; in dying child, 158-161; elective procedures, 158; in leukemia, 160

Oral care, of dying patient, 83; and emotional needs of patient, 77, 91; importance of, 20-21, 77; and maxillofacial prosthesis, 173-175; and need for good oral hygiene, 209; and need for programs to provide oral care to dying patient, 212; neurological aspects of, 99-105; with oral cancer, 208-213; with oral manifestations, 208-213; parenteral feeding, 103-104; and patient's position, 102; philosophy for, 16-23; and prosthodontic care decisions, 173; and role of dental hygienist, 20, 22; and role of dentist, 18, 20, 22; and role of nurse, 20, 22; and role of physician, 18, 20, 22; and self-care vs. dependency, 210

Oral care, of terminally ill cancer child, 150-155; oral hygiene, 150-151; oral side effects of drug therapy, 150

Oral care, of terminally ill patient, vii, ix, 179-181; and alcohol ingestion, 45; carotid body syndrome, 43; curative surgery, 47; during disease remission, 165-166; and disease severity, 47-49; drooling, 42-43; drug interaction, 46; elective procedures, 34; infection, 38; irradiation osteonecrosis, 35-36; irradiation therpay, 47; management of, 34-51; nutrition, 44-45; odor, 37-38; oral hygiene, 34; oral irrigation, 40-42; oxygen therapy, 45; pain management, 36; palliative therapy, 47; and philosophy for, 33-34; and psychological care, 50; and psychological effects of, 163; and smoking, 45; xerostomia, 39-40; *see also* Dentist; Oral hygiene; Stomatitis; Xerostomia

Oral dehydration, 159

Oral disease: causes of, 77-91; and dystonic syndrome, 119; psychological fears in, 90-91; as side effect of drug therapy, 114; therapy of, 84-87, 91; *see also* Dying patient

Oral gratification, *see* Mouth

Oral hygiene: importance of in patients receiving antitumor agents, 111; in oral cancer therapy, 28-30; in postoperative oral cancer patient, 192; procedures in oral cancer care, 163-164, 165-166; and role of dentist, 163

Oral hygiene, of dying patient, 77, 85, 9; effect of cardio-pulmonary disturbances on, 90; effect of gastrointestinal disturbances on, 90; role of dental hygienist in, 20; role of dental team in, 20; role of nurse in, 20

Oral hygiene, of terminally ill patient, 167; movie film concerning, 168; procedures in, 167-170; *see also* Dental care

Oral infection, in dying patient, 77, 82-85; bacterial, 84; causes of, 83-84; diptheroid, 83; and drug therapy, 84; manifestations of, 82; oral monilial, 83; proteus, 83; staphylococci, 83; streptococci, 83; and

surgery, 84; susceptibility to, 84, 89; treatment of, 82-85
Oral infections, treatment of in children, 159
Oral irrigation, 40-42
Oral moniliasis, 29, 38, 83, 161, 186; susceptibility to in patients receiving antitumor agents (i.e., cancer chemotherapy), 111; nonmonilial infections, 83
Oral prosthesis (e.g., intra-oral obturator), use of in postoperative period, 192
Orbital exenteration (patient), 193
Oropharyngeal cancer, 33, 37
Osmefar, 38
Osteoradionecrosis, 35-36, 38, 86; prevention of, 170
Ovarian cancer, and effectiveness of chemotherapy in, 109
Overeating, as oral gratification, 157
Overprotectiveness: of dying patient, 166; of oral cancer patient by family, 194
Oxazepam, 126
Oxygen therapy, 45
Oxygen transport, 90
Oxytetracycline, as cause of thrombocytopenia, 89
Ozena, 40
Pain: alteration in reaction to, 146, 147-148; caused by exposed dentin of tooth root and management of, 169-170; caused by gastrointestinal disturbances, 90; control of, 29-30; and narcotic addiction, 30; severity of, 146; sources of, 30; use of narcotic analgesics in relief of, 146, 147-148; use of phenothiazines in relief of, 147-148; see also Morphine; Pain; Pain, in dying patient
Pain, in dying child, 157, 159-160; meaning of, 157
Pain, in dying patient, 85-87; causes of, 86, 87; control of, 86, 87; drug therapy of, 86; individual variability in response to, 85; intractable, and control of, 87; and psychological fears in, 85, 86, 87; and reaction to, 87; and sensitivity to, 85; severity of, 85, 86, 87
Pain, in oral cancer, management of, 36-38; see also Pain, in dying patient
Pancreatic nuclease, 160
Pantopon, 37
Paramedical aides, role of in patient's final days, 49
Paranoia, in postoperative patient, 59, 60
Paraplegic patient, oral care of, 168
Paredrine hydrobromide, 43
Parenteral feeding, of dying patient, 79, 103-104
Parents, of dying child: and care of dying child, 157-158; and elective procedures, 158
Pargyline, 130
Parnate, 46; see also Tranylcypronine
Pastor, role of with oral cancer patients, 228-232
Pastoral care, of oral cancer patients, 228-232
Patient: see other entries in Index
Patient, dying, see Dying patient
Patient care: role of nurse in, 195-207; supportive therpay, 198
Patient-family relationships, and effect on oral tissues, 91
Penicillin: as cause of anemia, 88; oral complications of, 186; in treatment of infection in oral cancer patient, 85
Pentazocine, see Talwin
Percodan, 36
Peretz, David, 68-74
Periodontal disease, in dying patient, 86
Periodontics, 179
Periodontitis, in dying patient, 77
Peripheral nerve interruption, and control of pain, 30

Peripheral neurotomy, in control of intractable pain in oral cancer, 87
Periwinkle plant, 108
Pettit, Helen, viii
Pharmacotherapeutics, role of in thanatology, 143
Phenacetin, as cause of anemia, 88
Phenelzine, 130
Phenergan, 87; *see also* Promethazine
Phenobarbital, as cause of thrombocytopenia, 89
Phenothiazines, use of in pain relief, 147-148
Phenothiazine derivatives, 115-121; contraindications, 120-121; drug interactions, 120-121; indications for, 116; and "oral syndrome," 118; pharmacological effects of, 116-120, 126; side effects of, 117-120; *see also* "Major tranquilizers"
Phenylbutazone: and association with leukopenia, 89; as cause of thrombocytopenia, 89
Physician: and euthanasia, 49; and drug treatment of oral cancer patient, 143-149; and drug treatment of terminal patient, 143-149; and responsibility for care of dying patient, 155; role of, 52; role of in care of dying patient, 24-30, 91; role of in care of family of dying patient, 24, 27; role of in care of geriatric patient, 188; role of in oral care of patient, 20; role of in patient's final days, 49-50; *see* other entries
Platelet transfusions, in treatment of thrombocytopenia, 89-90
Pneumonia, 83
Pontocaine spray, 37
Post-irradiated teeth, 33
Postoperative nursing, oral cancer care: complications, 193; procedures, 190-194; role of nurse, 190-194
Postoperative psychological states of cancer patient, 58-61; anxiety, 59; counterphobia ("bravado behavior"), 60; depression, 59; hostility, as projected anger, 59; hypochondriasis, 59; obsessive compulsive reactions, 60; regression to dependency of childhood, 58; schizophrenia or postoperative panic, 60
Postoperative radiation, of intra-oral cancer patient, 191
Potassium chloride, 118
Potassium iodide, 39
Prednisone, in treatment of thrombocytopenic purpura, 89
Prefrontal leucotomy, and control of pain, 30
Prichard, Elizabeth R., 214-227
Pro-Banthine, 82
Procaine amide, and association with leukopenia, 89
Prochlorperazine, in control of vomiting, 90; contraindications of, 90; side effects of, 90
Project CAM (Crisis Awareness and Management), 201-202
Promethazine, 120, 122
Prostate cancer, and effectiveness of chemotherapy in, 109
Prosthodontic care, of oral cancer patient: decision to provide care, 173; and life expectancy of patient, 173-175; problems involved in, 173; *see also* Oral prosthesis
Prosthodontist, and dying patient, 173; responsibility of, 175
Protein hydrolysates, *see* Amigen
Protein loss, in cachexia, 77
Protein synthesis, 78
Protenium, 78
Proteus infection, in oral cancer patient, 83
Psychological care, of dying oral cancer patient, 50
Psychological reactions, of family to news of a fatal illness, 57-58
Psychological reactions, of patient: abandonment, 57; fear, 56-57; postoperative, 58-61

Psychopharmacoligical agents, 112-142; mechanisms of action, 113; side effects of, 113-115; use of in care of dying patient, 113-142; use of in care of oral cancer patient, 143-149; use of in care of terminal patient, 143-149; use of incontrol of pain in oral cancer; *see also* Antidepressants; Anxiolytic sedatives; Neuroleptic agents; Psychostimulants; *see* specific drug names
Psychoses, drug therapy for, 115
Psychosocial aspects, of oral care in dying patient, 3-15
Psychostimulants, 113
Psychotic depression, and bereavement, 71
Psychotherapy, in pain management of dying patient, 37
Purpura, and thrombocytopenia, 89
Pyelonephritis, 84
Pyocyanosis infection, 193
Quigley, M. B., 167-172
Radiation necrosis of bone, as side effect of radiation therapy, 53
Radiation therapy, in oral cancer patient, 53; side effects of, 53
Radiotherapist, relationship to dying patient, 92-98; and family, 93
Radiotherapy: recovery from, 78; complications of, 86, 88, 89
Rationalization, as adaptive mechanism to cope with loss, 70
Reeves, Robert B., Jr., 228-232
Regression: as adaptive mechanism to cope with loss, 70; as response to death, 71
Rejection, of terminally ill child, 152
Remission of disease, and dental care, 165-166
Reserpine, 120
Respaire, *see* Acetylcysteine
Respiratory depressants: Demerol, 147; morphine, 147
Responsibility for care of dying patient, of physician, 155
RNA synthesis, 108

Rubber bite block, use of in oral hygiene, 169
"Safe conduct," 14
St. Christopher's Hospice, and management of dying patient, 8
Salicylates, as cause of thrombocytopenia, 89
Saline, in care of oral cancer patient, 164
Sarcoma, and effectiveness of chemotherapy in, 109
Saunders, Cicely, 8
Schaaf, Norman G., 173-177
Scheman, Paul, 162-166
Schizophrenia, 113
Schizophrenia, or postoperative panic, drug treatment of, 60
Schoenberg, Bernard, 3-15, 143-149
Seconal, 147
Sedative-hypnotic agents, 128, 135
Sedatives, in control of pain in oral cancer, 87
Sedatives-hypnotics: use of in care of oral cancer patient, 143-146; use of in care of terminal patient, 143, 146
Self-care of terminal patient, benefits of, 12
Self-confidence, in oral cancer patient, 193
Self-image, of dying patient, maintenance of, 223-224; *see also* Body-image; Disfigurement
Self-sufficiency, importance of in oral cancer patient, 193
Semicoma, and oral care in, 100
Serax, *see* Oxazepam
Shannon, I. L., 167-172
Silicote skin protective spray or cream, 43
Sinequan, 49
Smoking: and oral care of dying patient, 45; as oral gratification, 157
Smoking, in oral cancer patient, 54-55; psychological fears involved, 54
Social work: reality focus of, 215, 217; responsibility of, 218, 226

Social worker: as part of interdisciplinary team, 224; and relationship with patient and family, 220-224; role of in bereavement, 225-226; role of in care of dying patient, 210-212, 214-227; role of in care of family of dying patient, 216, 217-219, 225
Soma, see Carisoprodol
Squamous cell carcinoma, 86
Squamous cell epithelioma, 109
Staff conferences, 199
Stannous fluoridegel, use of in oral hygiene, 168, 169, 170
Staphylococci infection, in oral cancer patient, 83
Stomatitis, as side effect of cancer chemotherapy, 110
Stomatitis medicamentosa, 119, 125
Streptococci infection, in oral cancer patient, 83
Streptomycin: as cause of anemia, 88; as cause of thrombocytopenia, 89; in treatment of infection in oral cancer patient, 85
Suicide, 59
Sulfonamides: as cause of anemia, 88; as cause of thrombocytopenia, 89
"Supportive therapy," in working with dying patient, 198
Surfak capsules, 45
Surgery: alimentary tract decompression, 90; and disfigurement, 143; of dying patient, 91; of oral cancer patients, psychological effects of, 229-232; recovery from, 78; on sexual organs, psychological reactions to, 59; on urinary or rectal sphincters, psychological reactions to, 60; see also Disfigurement
Sustagen, as dietary supplement, 80
Tachycardia, 90
Tachypnea, 90
Talwin, 36
Tea, use of in control of pain in oral cancer, 86

Team approach, to care of dying patient: benefits of for dying patient, 200; benefits of for staff, 198-199; role of nurse in, 198-199; see also Medical team
Teeth capping, see Elective procedures
Terminal care: use of analgesic agents in, 143-149; use of psychopharmacological agents in, 143-149
Terminal care facility, 224
"Terminal condition, the," 16-17; degrees of terminus, 16
Terminal patient: oral hygiene in, 85; prevention of infection in, 85; prolonging life of, 85
Terminally ill patient: care facilities for, 224; and community resources, 224; dental care of, 167-170; and home care, 224-225; and nursing home, 224; oral care of, 179-181
Tetracycline, side effects of, 158
Tetracycline, in treatment of infection in oral cancer patient, 85
"Therapeutic use of self," in the care of dying patient, 196
Therapy, of oral cancer patient, see Dietary therapy; Fever; Hematologic complications; Infection; Oral cancer; Oral cancer, complications of; Pain; Pain, in oral cancer; Prosthodontic care, of oral cancer patient
Thioxanthene derivatives, 121; see also Phenothiazine derivatives
Thorazine, 87, 145; use of in control of pain in oral cancer, 86; use of in postoperative patient, 60
Thrombosis, and thrombocytopenia, 89
Thumb sucking, 157
Thymidylic acid, 108
Thyroid cancer, and effectiveness of chemotherapy in, 109
Thyrotoxicosis, and grief reaction, 68-69
Tincture of opium, 81

Tofranil, use of in control of pain in oral cancer, 86
Tongue depressor, padded, use of in oral hygiene, 169
Toothbrush, battery-driven, 168
Toothpaste: desensitizing, 169-170; ingestible, 168
Topical fluoride treatment, 82
Toxoplasmosis, 84
Tracheitis sicca, 193
Tracheostomy, 102; as cause of oral infection, 83
Tracheotomy, of oral cancer patient, 229-231; and communication, 229-230
Tranquilizers, 36; use of in terminal patient, 101; *see also* Antianxiety agents; Antipsychotic agents; individual drugs
Tranylcypromine, 130, 135
Tricyclic antidepressants, 128; drug interaction, 130; pharmacological effects of, 129; therapeutic use of, 128-129
Tube feeding, of dying patient, 79
Tuberculosis, and grief reaction, 68-69
Tybamate, 123
Uremic stomatitis, 160
Valium, *see* Diazepam
Varidase, 38
Veterans Administration Dental Service, Houston, Texas, 168

Vinca rosea, 108
Vincristine, 110
Visiting Nurse Association, 32, 225
Vitamin A, 82
Vitamin B complex, 78
Vitamin K substitutes, as cause of anemia, 88
Vomiting, caused by gastrointestinal disturbances, 90; control of, 90
Walter Reed Army Medical Center, Washington, D.C., 201
Water Pic, use of by terminally ill patient, 165
Water spray, use of in oral hygiene, 168
Weakness, in dying patient, 77
Weight loss, in dying patient, 77
White blood cell transfusion, as experimental technique in treatment of leukopenia, 89
Wilms tumor of the kidney, and effectiveness of chemotherapy in, 109
Wound healing, 78, 81
Xerostomia, 39-40, 41, 114, 118, 121, 122, 127, 131 187; in dying patient, 77, 82
Xylocaine ointment, 37; use of in control of pain in oral cancer, 86
Xylocaine viscous, 37; use of in control of pain in oral cancer, 86
Zinc peroxide packs, 192